# Perspectives on the Department of Defense Global Emerging Infections Surveillance and Response System

## *A Program Review*

Philip S. Brachman, Heather C. O'Maonaigh, and Richard N. Miller, *Editors*

Committee to Review the Department of Defense Global Emerging Infections Surveillance and Response System

Medical Follow-Up Agency

INSTITUTE OF MEDICINE

NATIONAL ACADEMY PRESS
Washington, D.C.

**NATIONAL ACADEMY PRESS • 2101 Constitution Avenue, N.W. • Washington, DC 20418**

NOTICE: The project that is the subject of this report was approved by the Governing Board of the National Research Council, whose members are drawn from the councils of the National Academy of Sciences, the National Academy of Engineering, and the Institute of Medicine. The members of the committee responsible for the report were chosen for their special competences and with regard for appropriate balance.

Support for this project was provided by Contract No. DAM17-00-P-0412. The views presented in this report are those of the Institute of Medicine Committee to Review the Department of Defense Global Emerging Infections Surveillance Response System and are not necessarily those of the funding agencies.

International Standard Book Number 0-309-07635-8

Additional copies of this report are available for sale from the National Academy Press, 2101 Constitution Avenue, N.W., Box 285, Washington, DC 20055. Call (800) 624-6242 or (202) 334-3313 (in the Washington metropolitan area), or visit the NAP's home page at **www.nap.edu.** The full text of this report is available at **www.nap.edu.**

For more information about the Institute of Medicine, visit the IOM home page at: **www.iom.edu.**



Printed in the United States of America.

The serpent has been a symbol of long life, healing, and knowledge among almost all cultures and religions since the beginning of recorded history. The serpent adopted as a logotype by the Institute of Medicine is a relief carving from ancient Greece, now held by the Staatliche Museen in Berlin.

*"Knowing is not enough; we must apply.
Willing is not enough; we must do."*

—Goethe

INSTITUTE OF MEDICINE

**Shaping the Future for Health**

# THE NATIONAL ACADEMIES

National Academy of Sciences
National Academy of Engineering
Institute of Medicine
National Research Council

The **National Academy of Sciences** is a private, nonprofit, self-perpetuating society of distinguished scholars engaged in scientific and engineering research, dedicated to the furtherance of science and technology and to their use for the general welfare. Upon the authority of the charter granted to it by the Congress in 1863, the Academy has a mandate that requires it to advise the federal government on scientific and technical matters. Dr. Bruce M. Alberts is president of the National Academy of Sciences.

The **National Academy of Engineering** was established in 1964, under the charter of the National Academy of Sciences, as a parallel organization of outstanding engineers. It is autonomous in its administration and in the selection of its members, sharing with the National Academy of Sciences the responsibility for advising the federal government. The National Academy of Engineering also sponsors engineering programs aimed at meeting national needs, encourages education and research, and recognizes the superior achievements of engineers. Dr. Wm. A. Wulf is president of the National Academy of Engineering.

The **Institute of Medicine** was established in 1970 by the National Academy of Sciences to secure the services of eminent members of appropriate professions in the examination of policy matters pertaining to the health of the public. The Institute acts under the responsibility given to the National Academy of Sciences by its congressional charter to be an adviser to the federal government and, upon its own initiative, to identify issues of medical care, research, and education. Dr. Kenneth I. Shine is president of the Institute of Medicine.

The **National Research Council** was organized by the National Academy of Sciences in 1916 to associate the broad community of science and technology with the Academy's purposes of furthering knowledge and advising the federal government. Functioning in accordance with general policies determined by the Academy, the Council has become the principal operating agency of both the National Academy of Sciences and the National Academy of Engineering in providing services to the government, the public, and the scientific and engineering communities. The Council is administered jointly by both Academies and the Institute of Medicine. Dr. Bruce M. Alberts and Dr. Wm. A. Wulf are chairman and vice chairman, respectively, of the National Research Council.

## COMMITTEE TO REVIEW THE DEPARTMENT OF DEFENSE GLOBAL EMERGING INFECTIONS SURVEILLANCE AND RESPONSE SYSTEM

**PHILIP S. BRACHMAN** (*Chair*), Professor, Department of International Health, Rollins School of Public Health, Emory University, Atlanta, Georgia

**RUTH L. BERKELMAN**, Professor, Department of Epidemiology, Rollins School of Public Health, Emory University, Atlanta, Georgia

**DONALD S. BURKE**, Professor, Department of International Health and Director of the Center for Immunization Research, Johns Hopkins School of Public Health, Baltimore, Maryland

**KATHLEEN F. GENSHEIMER**, State Epidemiologist, Bureau of Health, Maine Department of Human Services, Augusta, Maine

**C. JAMES HOSPEDALES**, Director, Caribbean Epidemiology Center, Pan American Health Organization, World Health Organization, Port of Spain, Trinidad, West Indies

**ANN MARIE KIMBALL**, Professor, Health Services and Epidemiology, Adjunct in Medicine, University of Washington, Seattle, Washington

**GUÉNAËL R. RODIER**, Director, Department of Communicable Disease Surveillance and Response, World Health Organization, Geneva, Switzerland

**RONALD K. ST. JOHN**, Executive Director, Center for Emergency Preparedness and Response, Health Canada, Ottawa, Ontario, Canada

*Project Staff*

**RICHARD N. MILLER,** Study Director
**HEATHER C. O'MAONAIGH,** Program Officer
**PAMELA RAMEY-McCRAY,** Administrative Assistant
**ANDREA COHEN,** Financial Associate

# Preface

The U.S. Department of Defense (DoD) has historically defined its interest in infectious diseases almost exclusively in terms of "battle-stopper" illnesses—those resulting in acute effects that can directly affect military operations. Although this approach remains central to the U.S. military's infectious disease doctrine, development of the DoD Global Emerging Infections Surveillance and Response System (GEIS) is part of an important transition in the way that the threat of infectious diseases—and, more specifically, the threat of emerging infectious diseases—is perceived and addressed by the U.S. military.

Emerging infectious disease surveillance is sustained globally through a network of activities maintained through the collective efforts of numerous governmental and nongovernmental agencies. It is through the contributions of many partners that surveillance for emerging infectious diseases is possible. The DoD possesses valuable resources that can be brought to bear in this effort. It maintains an extensive, diverse array of laboratory facilities, both within the United States and overseas. These DoD laboratories can perform routine diagnostic testing, but they also possess rare, sometimes unique, diagnostic capabilities. DoD overseas laboratories are located throughout the world in areas where the potential for the emergence of infectious diseases is high. Often, laboratories operate in regions where alternative laboratory resources are sparse or nonexistent (e.g., sub-Saharan Africa). No other organization or government in the world maintains such extensive or capable laboratory facilities and staffing internationally. DoD laboratory facilities represent medical research, public health, and diplomatic resources that serve U.S. military, U.S. civilian, and global interests alike.

For more than a decade, formal DoD participation in emerging infectious disease surveillance has been encouraged by many in the U.S. public health community and within the DoD. In 1996, Presidential Decision Directive NSTC-7 (NSTC is the National Science and Technology Council of the Executive Office of the President) transformed these recommendations into a mandate. Thereafter, the National Intelligence Council declared emerging infectious diseases to be a threat to the national security of the United States, underscoring the importance of DoD participation in disease surveillance efforts. This role is not an altogether new one, as the DoD has been conducting various infectious disease surveillance projects (e.g., for influenza) for many years. Accommodation of its expanded role has led the DoD to implement GEIS. The committee recognizes this effort as a responsive and effective step toward addressing the problem of emerging infectious diseases.

We would like to thank the staff of the DoD laboratories, both domestic and overseas, and the staff of the GEIS Central Hub for the time and effort that they have invested in sharing with us information about the GEIS operations that they support. This review effort was very much a collegial one, and the report benefited from the openness of all those who provided us with documentation, presentations, and conversations. This study was also enriched by the insights that GEIS collaborators and associates provided regarding their views of GEIS from the outside looking in. Lists of the laboratory staff and GEIS collaborators and associates who shared their time with the committee can be found at the ends of Chapters 2 through 7 of this report. Any omissions are strictly the result of oversight.

The support provided by Institute of Medicine staff was instrumental in keeping this study moving apace. We extend our thanks to Richard Miller, Heather O'Maonaigh, and Pamela Ramey-McCray of the Institute of Medicine's Medical Follow-Up Agency and to National Academies Travel staff, particularly Ann-Marie Walko, for their assistance. This study also benefited from the attention of Andrea Cohen, financial associate; Michael Hayes, consulting editor; and Linda Kilroy, contracting officer. Medical Follow-Up Agency staff members Phillip Bailey, Salem Fisseha, Lois Joellenbeck, and Karen Kazmerzak also helped along the way.

In addition, we are grateful to GEIS Central Hub staff members, particularly Joel Gaydos, Steve Gubenia, Patrick Kelley, Jennifer Rubenstein, and James Writer for their tireless assistance in preparing and compiling background documents and for helping to plan and negotiate the logistics of site visits. Likewise, we offer special thanks to Roxana Lescano, Lucy Rubio, and Trueman Sharp, Naval Medical Research Center Detachment,

Peru; Andrew Corwin and John Sisson, Naval Medical Research Unit 2, Indonesia; Gaye Ruble, Armed Forces Research Institute of Medical Sciences, Thailand; Cole Church, Naval Medical Research Unit 3, Egypt; Ronald Rosenberg, U.S. Army Medical Research Unit, Kenya; and Leslie Henry, Naval Health Research Center, San Diego, for their help in putting site visits together.

This report is a testament to the hard work, patience, and resolve of many. We extend to all involved our appreciation and gratitude.

Philip S. Brachman (*Committee Chair*)
Ruth L. Berkelman
Donald S. Burke
Kathleen F. Gensheimer
C. James Hospedales
Ann Marie Kimball
Guénaël R. Rodier
Ronald K. St. John

# Reviewers

This report has been reviewed in draft form by individuals chosen for their diverse perspectives and technical expertise, in accordance with procedures approved by the NRC's Report Review Committee. The purpose of this independent review is to provide candid and critical comments that will assist the institution in making its published report as sound as possible and to ensure that the report meets institutional standards for objectivity, evidence, and responsiveness to the study charge. The review comments and draft manuscript remain confidential to protect the integrity of the deliberative process. We wish to thank the following individuals for their review of this report:

**JAMES BANTA,** Adjunct Professor, International Public Health, International Health Policy, The George Washington University Medical Center
**KENNETH BART,** Director, Graduate School of Public Health, San Diego State University
**DAVID BRANDLING-BENNETT,** Deputy Director, Pan American Health Organization
**SCOTT HALSTEAD,** Adjunct Professor, Department of Preventive Medicine and Biostatistics, Uniformed Services University of the Health Sciences
**ROBERT HOLZMAN,** Professor of Clinical & Environmental Medicine, New York University School of Medicine
**JOSHUA LEDERBERG,** Raymond and Beverly Sackler Foundation Scholar, The Rockefeller University

**JAMES W. LEDUC,** Acting Director, Division of Viral and Rickettsial Diseases, National Center for Infectious Diseases, Centers for Disease Control and Prevention

**STEPHEN B. THACKER,** Assistant Surgeon General and Director, Epidemiology Program Office, Centers for Disease Control and Prevention

Although the reviewers listed above have provided many constructive comments and suggestions, they were not asked to endorse the conclusions or recommendations, nor did they see the final draft of the report before its release. The review of this report was overseen by Adel A. F. Mahmoud, President, Merck Vaccine Division, Merck & Co. Appointed by the National Research Council and Institute of Medicine, he was responsible for making certain that an independent examination of this report was carried out in accordance with institutional procedures and that all review comments were carefully considered. Responsibility for the final content of this report rests entirely with the authoring committee and the institution.

# Contents

# Acronyms and Abbreviations

| | |
|---|---|
| ADP | automated data processor |
| AFEB | Armed Forces Epidemiology Board |
| AFI | acute febrile illness |
| AFIERA | Air Force Institute for Environmental Safety and Occupational Health Risk Analysis |
| AFIP | Armed Forces Institute of Pathology |
| AFRIMS | Armed Forces Research Institute of Medical Sciences |
| AMREF | African Medical and Research Foundation |
| AFRESS | Air Force Reportable Events Surveillance System |
| AIDS | Acquired Immunodeficiency Syndrome |
| BSL | biosafety level |
| CAREC | Caribbean Epidemiology Center |
| CDC | Centers for Disease Control and Prevention (United States) |
| CHCS/CHCS II | Department of Defense Composite Health Care System (I and II) |
| CHPPM | Center for Health Promotion and Preventive Medicine |
| CINC | Commander-in-Chief, Unified Combatant Command |

| | |
|---|---|
| CISET | Committee on International Science, Engineering, and Technology |
| CRDA | Cooperative Research and Development Agreement |
| | |
| DoD | Department of Defense (United States) |
| DMS | Department of Medical Services |
| DMSS | Defense Medical Surveillance System |
| | |
| EID | emerging infectious disease |
| ELISA | enzyme linked immunosorbent assay |
| EMRO | Eastern Mediterranean Regional Office, World Health Organization |
| ENSO | El Niño/Southern Oscillation |
| EWORS | Early Warning Outbreak Response System |
| ESSENCE | Electronic Surveillance System for Early Notification of Community-Based Epidemics |
| | |
| FSN | foreign service national |
| FETP | Field Epidemiology Training Program |
| FLUNET | WHO's influenza surveillance system |
| | |
| GEIS | Global Emerging Infections Surveillance and Response System |
| GIS | geographic information system |
| GISP | Gonococcal Isolate Surveillance Project |
| | |
| HIV | Human Immunodeficiency Virus |
| | |
| ILRI | International Livestock Research Institute |
| IOM | Institute of Medicine |
| IT | information technology |
| IS | information systems |
| INS | Instituto Nacional de Salud (Peru) |
| | |
| JICA | Japanese International Cooperative Agency |
| | |
| KEMRI | Kenya Medical Research Institute |
| | |
| LITS | Laboratory Information Tracking System |
| | |
| MDR-TB | multi-drug-resistant tuberculosis |
| MEDCOM | Medical Command |
| MFO | U.S. Multinational Forces and Observers |

| | |
|---|---|
| MHS | Military Health System |
| MIDRP | Military Infectious Disease Research Program |
| MoH | Ministry of Health |
| MOHP | Ministry of Health and Population (Egypt) |
| MSF | Médicins Sans Frontières; Doctors without Borders |
| | |
| NAMRID | Naval Medical Research Institute Detachment |
| NAMRU-2 | Naval Medical Research Unit 2 |
| NAMRU-3 | Naval Medical Research Unit 3 |
| NASA | National Aeronautics and Space Administration |
| NDRS | Naval Disease Reporting System |
| NEHC | Naval Environmental Health Center |
| NEPMU | Navy Environmental and Preventive Medicine Unit |
| NHRC | Naval Health Research Center |
| NIAID | National Institute of Allergy and Infectious Diseases |
| NMRCD | Naval Medical Research Center Detachment |
| NGO | nongovernmental organization |
| NIH | National Institutes of Health |
| NSTC-7 | National Science and Technology Council, Executive Office of the President, Presidential Decision Directive NSTC-7 |
| NSDD | National Security Decision Directive |
| | |
| OGE | Oficina General de Epidemiologia (Ministry of Health Office of Epidemiology, Peru) |
| OSTP | Office of Science and Technology Policy |
| | |
| PACOM | Pacific Command |
| PAHO | Pan American Health Organization |
| PHLIS | Public Health Laboratory Information System |
| | |
| RSD | Research Sciences Department |
| | |
| SEATO | Southeast Asia Treaty Organization |
| SOUTHCOM | Southern Command |
| STD | sexually transmitted disease |
| | |
| TAML | Theater Area Medical Laboratory |
| TB | tuberculosis |
| TEPHINET | Training in Epidemiology and Public Health Intervention Network |
| TMA | Tricare Management Area |

| | |
|---|---|
| USAID | United States Agency for International Development |
| USAID-VIGIA | United States Agency for International Development–project Addressing Threats of Emerging and Re-emerging Infectious Diseases |
| USAMRIID | United States Army Medical Research Institute of Infectious Diseases |
| USAMRU-K | United States Army Medical Research Unit, Kenya |
| U.S. CDC | United States Centers for Disease Control and Prevention |
| USUHS | United States Uniformed Services University of the Health Sciences |
| VEE | Venezuelan Equine Encephalitis |
| VIGIA | Addressing Threats of Emerging and Re-Emerging Infectious Diseases project |
| VPHL | Virtual Public Health Laboratory |
| VOIP | Voice Over Internet Protocol |
| VSAT | very small apperature terminal |
| WHO | World Health Organization |
| WRAIR | Walter Reed Army Institute of Research |

# GEIS Maps

Source: J. Writer, Department of Defense Global Emerging Infections Surveillance and Response System.

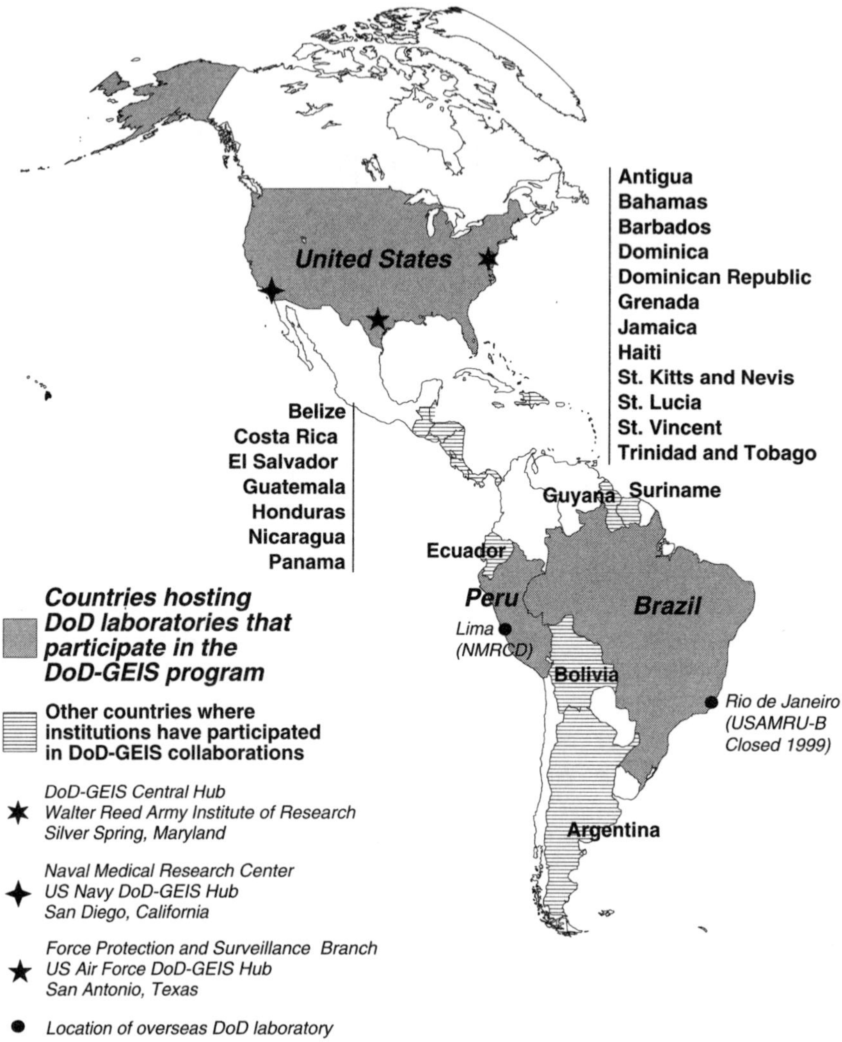
United States
Antigua
Bahamas
Barbados
Dominica
Dominican Republic
Grenada
Jamaica
Haiti
St. Kitts and Nevis
St. Lucia
St. Vincent
Trinidad and Tobago
Belize
Costa Rica
El Salvador
Guatemala
Honduras
Nicaragua
Panama
Guyana
Suriname
Ecuador
Peru
Brazil
Lima (NMRCD)
Bolivia
Rio de Janeiro (USAMRU-B Closed 1999)
Argentina
Countries hosting DoD laboratories that participate in the DoD-GEIS program
Other countries where institutions have participated in DoD-GEIS collaborations
DoD-GEIS Central Hub
Walter Reed Army Institute of Research
Silver Spring, Maryland
Naval Medical Research Center
US Navy DoD-GEIS Hub
San Diego, California
Force Protection and Surveillance Branch
US Air Force DoD-GEIS Hub
San Antonio, Texas
Location of overseas DoD laboratory

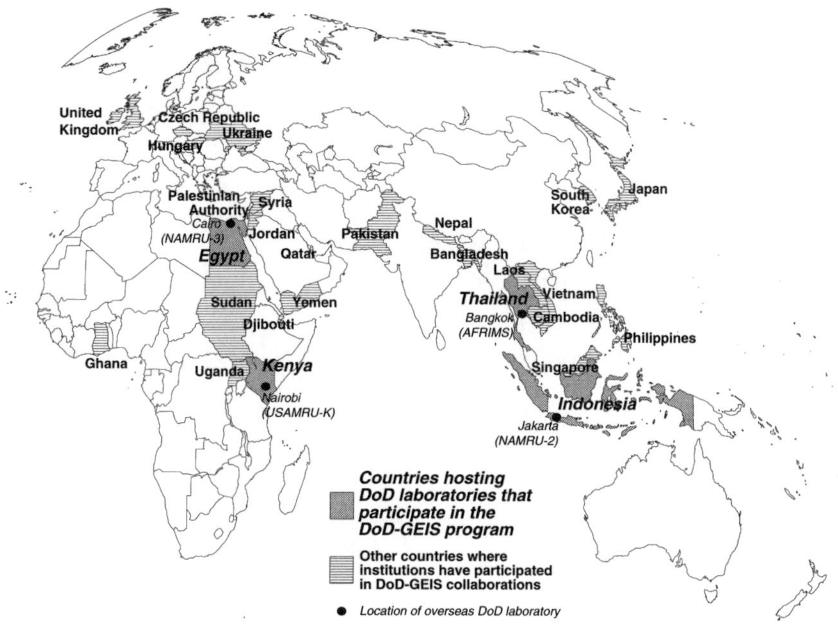
United Kingdom
Czech Republic
Ukraine
Hungary
Palestinian Authority
Syria
Cairo (NAMRU-3)
Jordan
Egypt
Qatar
Pakistan
Nepal
Bangladesh
South Korea
Japan
Laos
Thailand
Vietnam
Bangkok (AFRIMS)
Cambodia
Philippines
Sudan
Yemen
Djibouti
Ghana
Uganda
Kenya
Nairobi (USAMRU-K)
Singapore
Indonesia
Jakarta (NAMRU-2)
Countries hosting DoD laboratories that participate in the DoD-GEIS program
Other countries where institutions have participated in DoD-GEIS collaborations
Location of overseas DoD laboratory

# Executive Summary

In the years following World War II, the successful development and use of vaccines and antibiotics led to speculation that infectious diseases were vanquished foes. Defying these predictions, infectious diseases continue to be a leading cause of morbidity and mortality globally. In the 1980s, recognition of the devastating global epidemic of human immunodeficiency virus infection/AIDS focused the attention of the public and the public health community on the issue of emerging infectious diseases. Between 1987 and 1992, the Institute of Medicine (IOM) released three reports collectively urging improvements in the public health infrastructure in place nationally and internationally to address infectious diseases. The 1992 report, *Emerging Infections: Microbial Threats to Health in the United States* (IOM, 1992), was particularly instrumental in focusing attention on the threat of infectious disease emergence.

These concerns spurred a number of national and international initiatives, including the development of a Centers for Disease Control and Prevention (CDC) strategic plan for addressing emerging infectious diseases, a World Health Organization (WHO) resolution calling for strengthened infectious disease surveillance and response capabilities, and a formative National Science and Technology Council (NSTC) report. In 1996, the Executive Office of the President issued Presidential Decision Directive NSTC-7 (NSTC, 1996), which declared that national and international capabilities for infectious disease surveillance, prevention, and response were inadequate to protect the health of U.S. citizens from emerging infectious diseases and which called for a more robust national policy to improve these capabilities. NSTC-7 directed many U.S. federal agencies to take action and provided the following direction to the U.S. Department of Defense (DoD) (NSTC, 1996, pp. 4–5):

> The mission of the DoD will be expanded to include support of global surveillance, training, research, and response to emerging infectious disease threats. DoD will strengthen its global disease reduction efforts through: centralized coordination, improved preventive health programs and epidemiologic capabilities; and enhanced involvement with military treatment facilities and overseas laboratories.
>
> DoD will ensure the availability of diagnostic capabilities at its three domestic and six[1] overseas laboratories, using existing DoD resources. DoD will make available its overseas laboratory facilities, as appropriate, to serve as focal points for the training of foreign technicians and epidemiologists. If necessary, DoD will seek Chief of Mission concurrence to raise personnel ceilings at overseas laboratories, in accordance with NSDD [National Security Decision Directive]-38 procedures.

Since NSTC-7 was issued, U.S. agencies and international partners have taken many steps to achieve the goals of the directive and, more generally, to address global emerging infectious disease priorities. The DoD Global Emerging Infections Surveillance and Response System (GEIS) embodies the DoD's response to Presidential Decision Directive NSTC-7.

GEIS was established in 1997 by the assistant secretary of defense for health affairs, in response to NSTC-7, to serve as the focal point for DoD efforts to address emerging infectious diseases. In fiscal year 2001, funding for GEIS is expected to total approximately $8 million.[2] GEIS's annual budget is projected to increase over the next several years—to $9 million in fiscal year 2002, $10 million in 2004, and $11 million in 2005 (Kelley, 2000a). GEIS is a triservice program, and its activities are implemented within all three branches (Army, Navy,[3] and Air Force) of the armed forces, although GEIS has no direct command authority over the facilities that implement its activities. GEIS operates predominantly within the five currently operating Army and Navy overseas medical research laboratories and the infrastructure of the military health system (MHS). GEIS is managed by a Central Hub office located at the Walter Reed Army Institute of Research. The MHS[4] network of clinical and laboratory resources

[1]At the time that NSTC-7 was issued, the DoD operated six medical research laboratories overseas. In 1999, one laboratory (in Brazil) closed. At the time of this review, five DoD medical research laboratories are operating overseas.

[2]Excludes salaries for uniformed services personnel.

[3]Medical support for and public health surveillance of Marine Corps personnel are provided by the Navy.

[4]For the sake of brevity, the committee uses the term "military health system," as does GEIS, to describe the clinical, nonclinical/research based (excluding the overseas laborato-

provides infrastructure important for GEIS. Within the MHS, the emphasis of GEIS is on the strengthening of laboratory-based surveillance, particularly for influenza and other respiratory illnesses, for reportable illnesses, for changes in antibiotic resistance patterns, and for other evidence of emerging infections. DoD overseas laboratories provide forward sites for GEIS activities. At overseas laboratories, GEIS's focus is primarily on sentinel surveillance of indigenous and expatriate populations for specific infectious disease target areas, or "pillars," specifically: influenza, drug-resistant enteric organisms, drug-resistant malaria, and febrile illnesses, including dengue.

## THE STUDY

The committee that prepared this report, the Committee to Review the Department of Defense Global Emerging Infections Surveillance and Response System, was convened at the request of GEIS management to evaluate the progress of the nascent GEIS. This committee's task was defined as follows:

The committee will assess the extent to which the strategic plans of the five Department of Defense Global Emerging Infections System laboratories appropriately address the surveillance needs for the identification and tracking of emerging infectious disease in their respective locations. Specific questions to be addressed by the committee are:

a. How well does each plan meet the minimal infectious disease surveillance requirements as prescribed in Presidential Decision Directive NSTC-7 and the DoD Strategic Plan?

b. How well do the laboratory programs agree with the approach to emerging infection surveillance espoused in the IOM report on emerging infections and the Centers for Disease Control and Prevention (CDC) national strategic plan?

c. How well do the laboratories meet the World Health Organization and/or CDC standards for evaluating surveillance systems making reasonable allowances for 1) the need to balance the interests of the host country against those of DoD and the U.S., and 2) the varying governmental infrastructures in the different countries?

---

ries), and field/deployable laboratories, as well as the military treatment facilities, which are a part of the military health system and within which GEIS is implemented. The committee recognizes that this distinction is somewhat simplistic, but considers it is a necessary distinction to make in discussing spheres of GEIS operation.

d. How well does each strategic plan respond to the particular infectious disease surveillance challenges and the cultural dictates extant in the region in which it is to be implemented?

e. How well are the laboratories working on the other goals of GEIS (response, training and capacity building, and research) in support of their surveillance activities?

The committee will also assess:

f. How well are GEIS program goals, objectives, and activities being carried out domestically; namely, within the military health system (MHS) and the GEIS Central Hub?

The committee's charge left room for interpretation regarding a number of its tasks. In particular, the committee interpreted its charge as intending review of all information available, including, but not limited to, overseas laboratory strategic planning documents. Also, the committee focused its review on the development of conclusions and recommendations with long-term, program-level relevance rather than on evaluating specific GEIS projects. The committee used WHO and CDC guidelines as reference tools in conducting this review. Discussion of the committee's approach to addressing its charge and additional background information regarding GEIS are presented in detail in Chapter 1, this report's introduction.

As part of this review, members of the committee visited Naval Medical Research Center Detachment, Peru; Naval Medical Research Unit 2, Indonesia; the Armed Forces Research Institute of Medical Sciences, Thailand; Naval Medical Research Unit 3, Egypt; the U.S. Army Medical Research Unit, Kenya; the Naval Health Research Center,[5] San Diego, California; and the U.S. Army Medical Research Institute of Infectious Diseases, Washington, D.C. It was not practical to visit all MHS sites that host GEIS-funded projects. Instead, the committee relied heavily on written documents and on summary presentations from and discussions with DoD personnel and collaborators to gain an understanding of GEIS efforts within the MHS and the Central Hub.

Chapters 2 through 7 of this report present the committee's assessments of GEIS implementation at overseas laboratories, at sites within the infrastructure of the MHS, and through the GEIS Central Hub. Each chapter contains distinct conclusions and recommendations. Chapter 8 of this

[5]During this trip, the committee also visited Navy Environmental and Preventive Medicine Unit 5 and the U.S. Naval Hospital, San Diego.

report presents summary conclusions and recommendations regarding GEIS as a whole. These summary recommendations are excerpted and presented here, in the Executive Summary, as well. The boxes at the end of this chapter provide, in brief, recommendations regarding the implementation of GEIS at the overseas laboratories, within the infrastructure of the MHS, and through the Central Hub. The recommendations that are presented in boxes in this chapter are discussed in greater detail elsewhere in this report (Chapters 2 through 7). Recommendations by their very nature focus on areas of program implementation where there exists room for improvement. For a more complete picture of GEIS and its component DoD partners—members of the "GEIS consortium"—readers are encouraged to refer to Chapters 1 through 8 of this report.

## SUMMARY CONCLUSION[6]

GEIS is an appropriate DoD response to Presidential Decision Directive NSTC-7 and to the threat posed to national security by emerging infectious diseases. The goals of GEIS are in U.S. military, U.S. civilian, and global health interests. GEIS, still in the early stages of development, has made substantial progress toward achieving its goals. With increased support, and some refinements, the program has the potential to meet and exceed the expectations of Presidential Decision Directive NSTC-7.

## SUMMARY RECOMMENDATIONS[7]

- GEIS is a critical and unique resource for the United States in the context of global affairs. It is the only U.S. entity that is devoted to infectious diseases globally and that has broad-based laboratory capacities in overseas settings. GEIS goals, as outlined in its strategic plan, *Addressing Emerging Infectious Disease Threats: A Strategic Plan for the Department of Defense* (GEIS, 1998), address the areas of mission expansion that NSTC-7 mandates (NSTC, 1996). GEIS has the potential to meet and even exceed the expectations of Presidential Decision Directive NSTC-7 in its implementation. To date, significant progress has been made toward meeting the goals of the program. The committee notes that investment in GEIS is small compared to the challenge of emerging infectious diseases. Consideration should be given to increasing DoD investment in GEIS to a level at which GEIS can have a more substantial impact internationally. The GEIS budget is quite small compared to the budgets of those agencies and programs with which GEIS seeks to partner.

---

[6]Summary conclusions are presented in greater detail in Chapter 8.

[7]Summary recommendations in this section are explained in greater detail in Chapter 8.

It is important, however, to keep in mind that GEIS was created by appending programmatic requirements onto existing DoD bases of operation. The continued success of GEIS is predicated on the availability of resources, through GEIS and others, sufficient to support the facilities that host GEIS and on the ability of those facilities to balance the demands of multiple stakeholders. Research and public health surveillance missions are of critical importance to the DoD and are essential to national security. Emerging infectious disease surveillance is an important part of DoD capacity to assess potential threats to the health of U.S. forces. Research and public health surveillance missions can be balanced so that they are mutually beneficial.

GEIS would also benefit from the expansion of the DoD facilities available to support it. Increased capacity within existing facilities and creation of additional laboratories in areas of high biodiversity and in other regions of the world where there is strong potential for infectious diseases to emerge would benefit GEIS surveillance efforts. The committee recognizes that to respond to the recommendations in this report and to fulfill the mission of the GEIS program, a considerable increase in funding and personnel resources will be required.

**Recommendation: Support for GEIS and the facilities that sustain it should be increased to allow GEIS to completely fulfill its potential.**

• If GEIS is to be of optimal benefit, its mission will need to be fully understood, accepted, and balanced against the needs and resources of other DoD laboratory stakeholders. To work in tandem with others, GEIS must function smoothly as a program. If GEIS is to work as a cohesive program, it is important that its activities be well coordinated within each laboratory, between laboratories, and with the Central Hub. At some facilities that are part of GEIS, a dedicated program manager has been designated to coordinate projects. This is a valuable approach and one that needs to be duplicated at all facilities to the extent possible. GEIS program managers need to possess expertise and experience in applied epidemiology and public health practice.

**Recommendation: The implementation of GEIS at all five overseas research laboratories and within the MHS service hubs should be coordinated by dedicated, on-site GEIS program managers who possess expertise and experience in applied epidemiology and the practice of public health.**

• Many of the facilities that are implementing GEIS projects lack an adequate number of staff possessing sufficient epidemiological expertise. As a result, some activities observed by the committee reflected incomplete incorporation of public health surveillance concepts. Infusion of epidemiological input can help ensure that GEIS concepts are clearly understood and that surveillance objectives are fully realized. The presence of a dedicated, on-site GEIS program manager who is well versed in public health and applied epidemiology is important, as mentioned above. Additional epidemiological input, on site and through the Central Hub, is also desirable.

**Recommendation: GEIS should take steps to increase the number of personnel possessing applied epidemiological expertise available on site at laboratory facilities and within the Central Hub.**

• Current GEIS infectious disease-related training efforts (e.g., the Overseas Medical Research Laboratory Orientation Training Program) are laudable, but they are modest relative to the needs of the DoD and its public health partners and to the potential contributions of GEIS. Training professionals (including foreign national public health workers and DoD personnel) to understand, monitor, control, and prevent emerging infections is an important goal of GEIS. Providing training opportunities for U.S. civilian scientists may also prove to be a valuable use of GEIS resources. Additional investments could be made to bolster existing GEIS training activities and to develop additional, structured training programs. Training needs to be coordinated among GEIS consortium members and needs to be conducted in collaboration with public health partners (e.g., other DoD entities, the CDC, governments that host overseas laboratories, international organizations [such as the WHO], academic institutions, the Training in Epidemiology and Public Health Intervention Network [TEPHINET], and others).

**Recommendation: GEIS's level of involvement in the training of DoD personnel, foreign national public health workers, and others should be increased.**

• Training is an extremely important but time-consuming GEIS goal. Current laboratory training activities appear to be largely project specific and do not appear to be closely coordinated within or between laboratories. Additional staffing is needed to effectively coordinate the training needs of DoD personnel, foreign national public health workers, and others.

**Recommendation: Facilities that support GEIS and that implement training programs should be staffed to accommodate their training needs.**

• Collaboration is necessary to ensure that GEIS activities succeed, and complement and support other efforts. GEIS is actively fostering collaboration and coordination with international partners and governmental agencies in partner countries. GEIS is also taking important steps to strengthen collaborations with U.S. partner agencies, but more needs to be done to formalize these partnerships. New partnerships and means of expanding and strengthening existing partnerships can be pursued even more actively. In particular, relationships with other U.S. agencies, such as the U.S. Agency for International Development (USAID) and the CDC, need to be expanded and more closely coordinated to encourage joint planning and shared project implementation with these agencies. GEIS needs to have an identity within the global public health community such that when new initiatives related to global infectious disease surveillance and response activities are being considered by governmental and non-governmental agencies, the potential usefulness of GEIS is considered by outside partners.

The committee notes that hiring foreign nationals to fill senior positions at overseas laboratories can benefit GEIS integration with host-country and international partners. The committee encourages the hiring of additional foreign service national personnel into senior-level positions where possible. Similarly, personnel assigned to the DoD from U.S. partner agencies, such as the CDC, the National Institutes of Health, universities, and state public health agencies, can help meet staffing needs while increasing DoD ties with those agencies. The committee endorses such arrangements and encourages GEIS to actively pursue them as a means of meeting DoD staffing needs.

**Recommendation: Pursuit of collaborative, well-coordinated relationships with international organizations, U.S. government agencies (including other DoD entities), and relevant agencies of foreign governments should be continued and expanded to the extent possible. As part of these collaborations, GEIS should encourage arrangements for the sharing of staff between U.S. and international partner agencies and DoD laboratory facilities.**

• It is important that mechanisms for rapidly communicating data and other information to public health partners positioned to take action in response to an infectious disease threat be clearly identified and used. Some DoD laboratories have evolved successful communications strategies, but these mechanisms do not appear to have developed as part of a cohesive GEIS plan.

**Recommendation: In consultation with the GEIS Central Hub and collaborators, GEIS sites should prepare and act on information dissemination plans that provide for the translation of information into timely public health action.**

• Centralized data collection and analysis (as appropriate) and routine reporting of GEIS data and other information are also needed. Current methods of disseminating GEIS information are important but are insufficient. Tools such as the GEIS website (GEISWeb) and the DoD Directory of Public Health Laboratory Services can be very useful communication resources. Production of a periodic GEIS-wide publication that synthesizes GEIS information (e.g., surveillance data, progress reports, and updates on new capabilities and accomplishments) may also be appropriate.

**Recommendation: Communication of surveillance and other information within the GEIS consortium, within the DoD, to public health partners, and to the public should be improved.**

• Many of the innovative systems and techniques that GEIS is developing or encouraging, such as the DoD Directory of Public Health Laboratory Services, the Early Warning Outbreak Response System, the Electronic Surveillance System for the Early Notification of Community-Based Epidemics, and numerous others, show great promise. It is important, however, that the need for new systems and techniques be thoroughly evaluated and that plans for system development and use be clearly defined (including identification of product developers with extensive relevant expertise and experience) before projects are undertaken. Prototype systems and techniques should also be systematically evaluated before they are put to widespread use. These steps are needed to ensure that new systems and techniques contribute optimally to GEIS, to the DoD, and to global emerging infectious disease surveillance efforts.

**Recommendation: Novel surveillance systems and techniques, though potentially an important part of GEIS, should be thoroughly evaluated and plans for their development and use should be clearly defined before substantial GEIS investments in their implementation are made.**

• Periodic external review can help to determine whether the goals of GEIS are being addressed and whether those goals remain appropriate.

**Recommendation: GEIS as a whole should be subject to periodic external review (every few years) to ensure that it remains focused on its goals and that its goals remain appropriate.**

• Apart from this formal, periodic program review process, it is also essential that GEIS management (i.e., the Central Hub) has available to it clear, consistent means of routinely receiving authoritative and timely management guidance from appropriate DoD authorities as well as a means of providing feedback to appropriate DoD authorities. It is also important that there be in place within the DoD command structure clear, consistent channels through which GEIS information can be reported to achieve timely action.

**Recommendation: Clear, consistent mechanisms for providing guidance to GEIS management and channels for the reporting of GEIS information within the DoD infrastructure should be in place.**

• The committee recognizes that managing a program as diverse and diffuse as GEIS is no small task. It appears to the committee that the Central Hub is limited in its ability to effectively coordinate GEIS by a lack of administrative authority and management resources. To ensure that project guidance is acted upon, GEIS management must be positioned so that it has the authority, as well as the responsibility, to affect GEIS project implementation.

**Recommendation: GEIS management authority should be commensurate with GEIS management responsibility if program objectives are to be effectively and efficiently met.**

• GEIS would benefit from a broader, more standardized project review process (to include use of structured proposal guidelines and timelines). Reviews need to incorporate input from various interested parties, such as partner agencies, overseas and MHS laboratory personnel, and other DoD representatives (e.g., Military Infectious Disease Research Program staff), as well as Central Hub staff. It may be useful to lengthen the project approval and funding cycle to allow projects to mature and to allow improved planning of new projects between reviews.

**Recommendation: Consideration should be given to revising the GEIS project review and approval process so that review and approval of GEIS projects is part of a more formally structured process—based on a set of guidelines and timelines that are clearly understood by GEIS consortium members—that includes input from individuals who represent various disciplines and interests.**

• Apart from the formal project review and approval process, Central Hub senior management staff need to make additional periodic visits to the respective laboratory facilities to provide project guidance and to assess needs for assistance and opportunities for collaboration. Increased guidance from the Central Hub may help to compensate for staffing deficiencies and can foster improved coordination of GEIS projects.

**Recommendation: Staffing levels permitting, overseas and MHS-based GEIS activities should receive additional periodic assessment and guidance from the GEIS Central Hub.**

**BOX 1-A**
**Recommendations That Are Repeated in Each Overseas Laboratory Evaluation**

DoD commitment to GEIS at overseas laboratories should be long term.

Consideration should be given to refining the focus of GEIS at the overseas laboratories to better enable diseases outside of the pillar areas to be addressed.

Consideration should be given to revising the current GEIS project application and review process.

Senior staff at overseas laboratories actively involved in GEIS projects should be conversant in the dominant language of the host country or should pursue, with the support of GEIS, language training, and should seek to become conversant to the extent possible.

**BOX 1-B**
**Chapter 2**
**Naval Medical Research Center Detachment, Peru (NMRCD)**

Full-time staff members should be assigned to NMRCD to meet staffing needs in the following areas:

- GEIS program management. The GEIS program manager should not have simultaneous responsibility for departmental management and administering overall NMRCD GEIS activities. The GEIS program manager should be full-time and on-site, and should possess, at a minimum, applied epidemiology and public health experience.
- Support for training activities. The coordination of training activities is an important but time-intensive GEIS task. This task should not be consigned to NMRCD department heads as a secondary responsibility.
- Epidemiology. Additional epidemiological support (including, but not necessarily limited to, a dedicated GEIS program manager) should be provided to help facilitate public health-oriented data analysis and study design and to provide a permanent link between NMRCD and the Oficina General de Epidemiologia (OGE) national surveillance system, as well as other public health partners.
- Administrative support. Extensive administrative requirements can impede the work of a scientific staff that is already stretched thin. Additional administrative (nonclerical) support should be provided so that NMRCD scientists can devote their talents to GEIS studies under way.

DoD and Peruvian training needs should be assessed formally, and the development of a structured NMRCD-hosted training program should be considered.

As GEIS project data are accumulated, they should be better used to supplement the OGE national surveillance system, provide early warnings of epidemics, and help guide public health responses.

NMRCD should take continued steps to maintain and enhance the multiple national and international partnerships that are necessary to fulfill the GEIS mission and to build national capacity in Peru.

**BOX 1-C**
**Chapter 3**
**Naval Medical Research Unit 2, Indonesia (NAMRU-2)**

The development of a structured NAMRU-2-hosted training program should be pursued.

As GEIS project data are accumulated, they should continue to be used to supplement the national surveillance system and should be better used to help guide public health response through improved sharing of information with international partners, such as the WHO and USAID.

NAMRU-2 should take continued steps to maintain and enhance the multiple national and international partnerships that are necessary to fulfill the GEIS mission and build national capacity in Indonesia.

NAMRU-2 should continue to support the development of the field laboratory in Cambodia.

The Early Warning Outbreak Response System should be evaluated for its capacity to serve as an early-warning system for the detection and investigation of epidemics and for the identification of new and novel pathogens before major investments in expanding the system are made.

**BOX 1-D**
**Chapter 4**
**Armed Forces Research Institute of Medical Sciences, Thailand (AFRIMS)**

As GEIS project data are accumulated, they should be better used to supplement national and regional surveillance systems and to help guide public health responses through improved reporting to authorities in the host country.

AFRIMS should continue to take steps to maintain and enhance the multiple national and international partnerships that are necessary to fulfill the GEIS mission.

AFRIMS GEIS efforts should be coordinated with the efforts of other DoD facilities (i.e., laboratories, the GEIS Central Hub, and other GEIS partners) that host GEIS projects in the region.

To fully realize GEIS objectives, AFRIMS should have a full-time, onsite GEIS program manager who possesses expertise in applied epidemiology and public health.

Influenza surveillance efforts should be coordinated with the Thai WHO collaborating laboratory.

The development of a structured AFRIMS-hosted training program should be considered.

**BOX 1-E**
**Chapter 5**
**Naval Medical Research Unit 3, Egypt (NAMRU-3)**

Additional applied epidemiological input should be provided to guide the development and conduct of NAMRU-3 GEIS projects to fully realize program goals.

Consideration should be given to obtaining a full-time, on-site manager possessing experience in applied epidemiology and public health for the GEIS program at NAMRU-3, or to providing more epidemiological and technical oversight responsibility to the manager of the Disease Surveillance Program, as the current NAMRU-3 organizational structure does not allow the Disease Surveillance Program to maximize collaboration and coordination of GEIS activities across the Research Sciences Department.

NAMRU-3 should ensure the long-term presence of foreign service national personnel to maximize the continuity of individual GEIS projects and provide the institutional memory and cultural sensitivity necessary for success of GEIS.

NAMRU-3, in coordination with the GEIS Central Hub, should expand partnerships with and continue to raise funds through (as applicable) sources such as USAID (country offices and its Global Bureau), the CDC (including FETP), the WHO, and other relevant agencies to the full extent possible to enhance in-country surveillance and response capacities.

NAMRU-3 should continue to support the Egyptian Ministry of Health and Population (MOHP) in gradually strengthening the MOHP's own capacity for surveillance across Egypt, with a particular focus on laboratory diagnostic capabilities. This support should also be extended to other countries of the region, resources permitting.

A comprehensive NAMRU-3 information plan that outlines the needs and mechanisms for the reporting of information to partners in public health activities and to the GEIS Central Hub should be developed and acted upon.

NAMRU-3 should actively pursue with its in-country partners resolution of issues regarding ownership of surveillance data and issues regarding the clearance of data for dissemination.

**BOX 1-F**
**Chapter 6**
**U.S. Army Medical Research Unit, Kenya (USAMRU-K)**

Current GEIS surveillance projects and activities should be continued, as they represent activities in support of the GEIS mission.

Expansion of the reach of GEIS activities should be considered.

USAMRU-K and the GEIS Central Hub should facilitate the acquisition of reagents for the diagnosis of Ebola, Marburg, Crimean-Congo, and Lassa hemorrhagic fevers (and other infectious disease entities, as applicable) to the extent possible.

Additional GEIS investment in improving USAMRU-K's laboratory capacity is needed and should be pursued, within program limits.

USAMRU-K should have a full-time GEIS program manager on site. The designated program manager should have training and expertise in applied epidemiology and public health.

The assignment of a CDC epidemiologist to USAMRU-K, the assignment of a military public health physician with epidemiological experience, or the assignment of a civilian medical epidemiologist with public health experience should be pursued. To fully realize the GEIS surveillance mission, there should be strong epidemiological input in USAMRU-K GEIS development and management.

USAMRU-K should explore the possibility of supplementing its military scientific staff with Kenyan nationals possessing comparable expertise to ensure continuity of projects, to expand expertise, and to foster collaborative relationships and project growth in important areas of public health surveillance.

The availability of staff with virological expertise within USAMRU-K would assist in the achievement of GEIS's goals and should be considered.

Collaborative relationships should continue to be forged and fostered to ensure that USAMRU-K is involved as a full partner in infectious disease surveillance and response activities.

DoD and Kenyan training needs should be assessed formally, and the development of a structured USAMRU-K-hosted training program should be considered.

In consultation with the GEIS Central Hub and public health partners, USAMRU-K should develop and implement a system for the dissemination of public health data in a routine and timely manner to ensure public health action.

Steps should be taken to link GEIS projects together as part of an integrated USAMRU-K GEIS effort.

Expansion and refined application of communications technologies should be pursued by USAMRU-K with GEIS support.

Effort should be directed to enhancement of the public health application of current geographic information system work (carried out in collaboration with the International Livestock Research Institute) so that such efforts can better result in information for action.

**BOX-2**
**Chapter 7**
**GEIS Central Hub and Military Health System Activities**

Staffing within the Central Hub should be increased so that its communication and coordination responsibilities can be optimally addressed.

The Central Hub should have available to it improved means of obtaining more and more frequent management guidance.

The Central Hub should be given more management authority so that it can successfully meet its objectives.

GEIS projects within the infrastructure of the MHS are important but should be more tightly integrated with each other and better coordinated with and supportive of activities conducted at the overseas laboratories.

GEIS efforts to build MHS public health laboratory capacity to detect and respond to emerging infectious diseases should be clearly focused and should be increased.

The development of new systems resources is an important goal of GEIS, but the needs and specifications for innovative surveillance systems and techniques should be clearly defined before they are undertaken, and caution should be used when implementing unproven systems and techniques on a large scale.

Central Hub-managed international capacity-building projects should be better coordinated with DoD laboratory facilities overseas and within the MHS, as appropriate.

Central Hub involvement in coordinating and supporting training activities relevant to emerging infectious disease surveillance and response should be increased.

The GEIS Central Hub should

Provide clear and specific guidance to laboratories regarding the goals of GEIS and the qualities that GEIS projects are expected to possess, actively assist laboratories in developing project plans, and provide periodic scientific guidance for projects under way, as needed.

Provide a mechanism for project review that is structured, that is clearly and consistently defined, that allows adequate time for project conduct between reviews, that results in timely feedback to the laboratories proposing projects, and that is carried out by a diverse panel of experts including Central Hub staff and others, such as senior DoD laboratory staff, Military Infectious Disease Research Program (MIDRP) staff, and other DoD and non-DoD representatives.

Consistently interact with staff directing GEIS projects to monitor project progress, evolving potential for collaboration, and needs for assistance.

Given personnel and other resource shortages, Central Hub conduct of surveillance projects is undesirable and should be minimized and avoided to the extent possible.

Improved means of centrally collecting, analyzing (as appropriate), and distributing surveillance data and other information in a timely manner need to be developed and implemented.

# 1

# Introduction

## BACKGROUND

In the years following World War II, the successful development and use of vaccines and antibiotics led to speculation that infectious diseases were vanquished foes (CDC, 1998; IOM, 1992, 2001; WHO, 1996, 2000c). Defying these predictions, infectious diseases continue to be a leading cause of morbidity and mortality globally (IOM, 2001; NIC, 2000; WHO, 2000c). Old scourges, such as tuberculosis, malaria, dengue, cholera, and influenza linger still. New challenges, such as human immunodeficiency virus (HIV) infection, multi-drug-resistant tuberculosis and other bacterial diseases, and various encephalitides and viral hemorrhagic fevers, have surfaced with grim frequency in recent years and are reminders that emerging and reemerging infectious diseases are threats worthy of continued concern and due vigilance.

In the 1980s, recognition of the devastating global HIV/AIDS epidemic focused the attention of the public and the public health community on the issue of emerging infectious diseases. Between 1987 and 1992, the Institute of Medicine (IOM) released three reports collectively urging improvements in the public health infrastructure in place nationally and internationally to address infectious diseases (IOM, 1987, 1988, 1992). The 1992 report, *Emerging Infections: Microbial Threats to Health in the United States*, was particularly instrumental in focusing attention on the threat of infectious disease emergence. These concerns spurred a number of national and international initiatives, including the development of a Centers for Disease Control and Prevention (CDC) strategic plan for addressing emerging infectious diseases (CDC, 1994), a World Health Organization (WHO) resolution calling for strengthened infectious disease surveillance and response capabilities (WHO, 1995), and a formative National Science and Technology Council Report (CISET, 1995).

In 1996, the Executive Office of the President issued Presidential Decision Directive NSTC-7 (NSTC is the National Science and Technology Council of the Executive Office of the President), which declared that national and international capabilities for infectious disease surveillance, prevention, and response were inadequate to protect the health of U.S. citizens from emerging infectious diseases and which called for a more robust national policy to improve these capabilities (NSTC, 1996). NSTC-7 directs U.S. federal agencies, namely, the U.S. Departments of Health and Human Services, State, Defense (DoD), Justice, Commerce, Agriculture, Interior, and Energy; the U.S. Agency for International Development; the National Aeronautics and Space Administration; the Environmental Protection Agency; the Intelligence Community; the White House Office of Science and Technology Policy; the National Security Council; the Domestic Policy Council; and the Office of Management and Budget to take action (NSTC, 1996). Responsibility for coordinating the multiagency response to the directive rests with the National Science and Technology Council Task Force on Emerging Infections (CISET, 1997; NSTC, 1996).

NSTC-7 provides the following direction to DoD (NSTC, 1996, pp. 4-5):

> The mission of the DoD will be expanded to include support of global surveillance, training, research, and response to emerging infectious disease threats. DoD will strengthen its global disease reduction efforts through: centralized coordination, improved preventive health programs and epidemiologic capabilities; and enhanced involvement with military treatment facilities and overseas laboratories.
>
> DoD will ensure the availability of diagnostic capabilities at its three domestic and six[1] overseas laboratories, using existing DoD resources. DoD will make available its overseas laboratory facilities, as appropriate, to serve as focal points for the training of foreign technicians and epidemiologists. If necessary, DoD will seek Chief of Mission concurrence to raise personnel ceilings at overseas laboratories, in accordance with NSDD [National Security Decision Directive]-38 procedures.

Since NSTC-7 was issued, U.S. agencies and international partners have taken many steps to achieve the goals of the directive and, more

[1]At the time that NSTC-7 was issued, the DoD operated six medical research laboratories overseas. In 1999, one laboratory (in Brazil) closed. At the time of this review, five DoD medical research laboratories are operating overseas.

generally, to address global emerging infectious disease priorities (CDC, 1998; CISET, 1997; DoS, 1999; GEIS, 1998; NIC, 2000; NIAID, 1996, 2000; USAID, 1998; WHO, 1996, 2000b). The DoD Global Emerging Infections Surveillance and Response System (GEIS) embodies the DoD response to Presidential Decision Directive NSTC-7.

## THE DEPARTMENT OF DEFENSE GLOBAL EMERGING INFECTIONS SURVEILLANCE AND RESPONSE SYSTEM

GEIS was established in 1997 by the assistant secretary of defense for health affairs, in response to NSTC-7, to serve as the focal point for "initiating and coordinating the identification, reporting and responding to emerging infectious disease problems" (Bancroft and Schlagel, 1997, p. 1) within the DoD. GEIS is a new program that supplements, but that does not replace, the ongoing research mission of DoD laboratories (Bancroft and Schlagel, 1997; Mazzuchi, 1999). GEIS was first allocated start-up funds in fiscal year 1997, although GEIS is officially considered to have begun in late 1998 (GEIS, 2001a). In fiscal year 2000, GEIS funding totaled $7 million (GEIS, 2000b). In fiscal year 2001, funding for GEIS is expected to total approximately $8 million (GEIS, 2000c).[2] GEIS's annual budget is projected to increase over the next several years—to $9 million in fiscal year 2002, $10 million in 2004, and $11 million in 2005 (Kelley, 2000a).

The U.S. Army is the designated executive agent for GEIS (Lister, 1997). GEIS is organizationally responsible to the Office of the Surgeon General of the U.S. Army (Martin, 1997c). GEIS is a triservice program, and its activities are implemented within all three branches (Army, Navy, and Air Force) of the armed forces, although GEIS has no direct command authority over the facilities that implement its activities. GEIS operates predominantly within the five currently operating Army and Navy overseas medical research laboratories and the infrastructure of the military health system[3] (MHS) (GEIS, 2000b). Within the MHS, GEIS has designated service hubs at the Naval Health Research Center, San Diego, California, and the U.S. Air Force Epidemiology Services Branch, Brooks Air Force Base, San Antonio, Texas, that serve as focal points for GEIS MHS

[2]Excludes salaries for uniformed personnel.

[3]For the sake of brevity, the committee uses the term "military health system" as does GEIS, to describe the clinical, nonclinical/research-based (excluding the overseas laboratories), and field/deployable laboratories, as well as the military treatment facilities, which are a part of the military health system and within which GEIS is implemented. The committee recognizes that this distinction is somewhat simplistic, but it is a necessary distinction to make in discussing spheres of GEIS operation.

Major organizations involved with DoD-GEIS

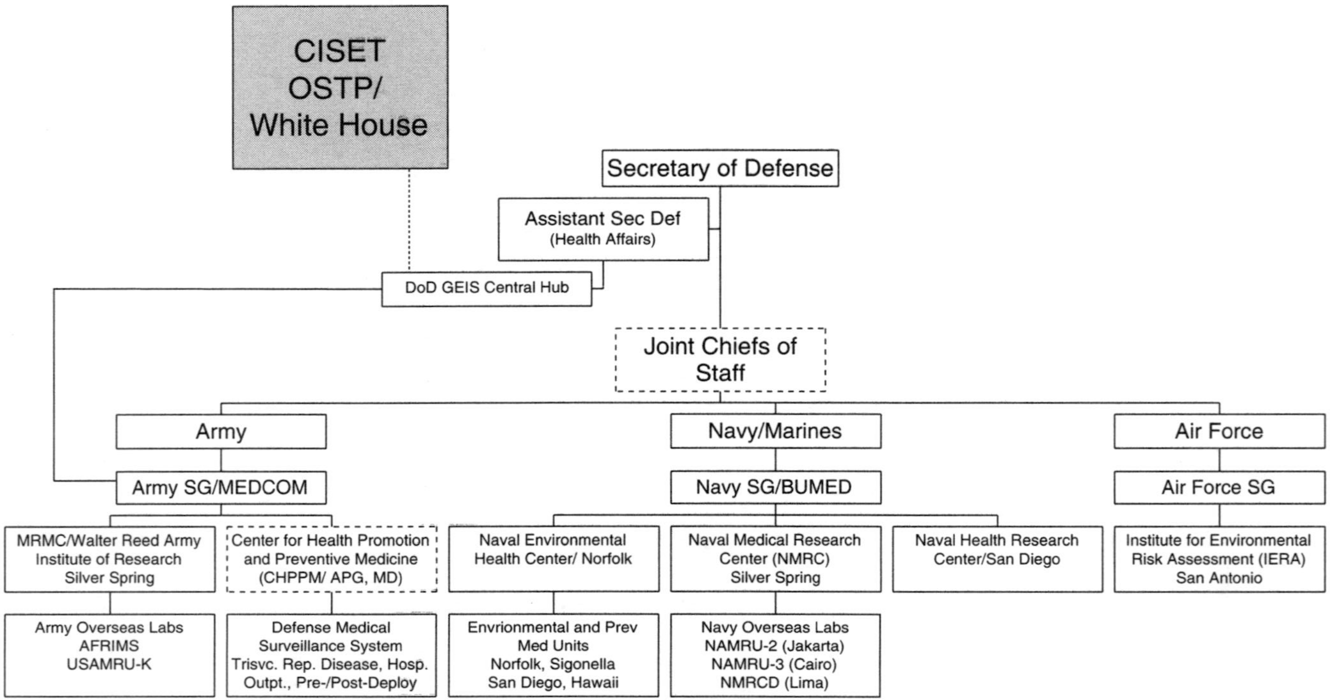


SOURCE: P. Kelley, Department of Defense Global Emerging Infections Surveillance and Response System.

activities (Gaydos, 1999). GEIS also collaborates with other components of the DoD, including the U.S. Army Medical Research Institute of Infectious Diseases (USAMRIID), Fort Detrick, Maryland; the Naval Environmental Health Center, Norfolk, Virginia; the U.S. Army Center for Health Promotion and Preventive Medicine, Aberdeen Proving Ground, Maryland; and other DoD sites within the United States and abroad. GEIS also provides support for and collaborates with non-DoD partners.

GEIS is managed by a Central Hub office that operates within and receives administrative support from the Walter Reed Army Institute of Research. Planning documents call for the Central Hub to be supported by a triservice staff (Bancroft and Schlagel, 1997), although no Air Force personnel are assigned to the Central Hub at present. The Central Hub is directed by a preventive medicine officer of the same service as the program's executive agent (the Army). GEIS receives periodic scientific input from the Armed Forces Epidemiology Board and periodic program management direction from a flag level[4] advisory board (Christopherson and Baldwin, 1997; Lister, 1997). GEIS occasionally receives non-DoD input as well, for example, through the Committee on International Science, Engineering, and Technology (CISET) (CISET, 1997) and through publicly attended GEIS symposia (GEIS, 1999b). In addition to providing GEIS program management, the Central Hub also directs surveillance, systems research, and capacity-building activities.

The MHS network of clinical and laboratory resources provides infrastructure and surveillance capabilities important for GEIS. Within the MHS, the emphasis of GEIS is on the strengthening of laboratory-based surveillance, particularly for influenza and other respiratory illnesses (GEIS, 1998), for reportable illnesses, for changes in antibiotic resistance patterns, and for other evidence of emerging infections.

Since the early 1900s, the DoD has maintained a network of medical research laboratory facilities overseas to help identify infectious diseases and to evaluate control measures (Gambel and Hibbs, 1996). These DoD overseas laboratories provide forward sites for GEIS activities. At present the DoD has five overseas laboratories, which are based in Lima, Peru; Jakarta, Indonesia; Bangkok, Thailand; Cairo, Egypt; and Nairobi, Kenya. In addition, these laboratories have field activities that operate in other nearby countries. The laboratory capacities that these facilities possess are often rare or unique within their regions of operation. GEIS was active in 38 countries in fiscal year 2000 (GEIS, 2000b). Many activities were directed through the overseas laboratories. At overseas laboratories, the focus of GEIS is primarily on the development of sentinel surveillance of indigenous and expatriate populations, as defined in its ambitious 1998

[4]General officer or admiral rank.

strategic plan, *Addressing Emerging Infectious Disease Threats: A Strategy for the Department of Defense* (GEIS, 1998).

The GEIS mission is centered around four goals that are similar to those of the CDC (CDC, 1994, 1998; GEIS, 1998). GEIS goals include the following (GEIS, 1998, p. 1):

> **Surveillance.** Detect and monitor emerging pathogens, the diseases they cause, and the factors influencing their emergence to protect military readiness, the health of DoD beneficiary populations, and other national interests.
>
> **Systems Research, Development, and Integration.** Integrate public health practices and improve capabilities in clinical medicine, military medicine, laboratory science, epidemiology, public health, and military medical research to facilitate the rapid identification and response to emerging infections
>
> **Response.** Enhance the prompt implementation of all prevention and control strategies for emerging infections to include improving communication of information about emerging agents.
>
> **Training and Capacity Building.** Leverage DoD and international public health infrastructures through training, networking, and other forms of assistance to support surveillance, assessment, response, and prevention of emerging infections.

These goals represent the organizing principles of GEIS activities carried out within the overseas laboratories, the infrastructure of the MHS, and the Central Hub—the constituent parts of the GEIS consortium (DoD partners in GEIS). GEIS has identified four "pillar" areas of infectious disease focus to guide surveillance efforts, particularly at overseas laboratories. Pillar areas are formally influenza, drug-resistant enteric organisms, drug-resistant malaria, and febrile illnesses, including dengue (GEIS, 1998). These target areas are intended to address a balance of disease areas that are important to the DoD, the U.S. population, and the international community, duly recognizing resource constraints.

## CHARGE TO THE COMMITTEE

This committee's task was defined as follows:

> The committee will assess the extent to which the strategic plans of the five Department of Defense Global Emerging Infections System laboratories appropriately address the surveillance needs for the identification and tracking of emerging infectious disease in their respective locations. Specific questions to be addressed by the committee are:

a. How well does each plan meet the minimal infectious disease surveillance requirements as prescribed in Presidential Decision Directive NSTC-7 and the DoD Strategic Plan?

b. How well do the laboratory programs agree with the approach to emerging infection surveillance espoused in the IOM report on emerging infections and the Centers for Disease Control and Prevention (CDC) national strategic plan?

c. How well do the laboratories meet the World Health Organization and/or CDC standards for evaluating surveillance systems making reasonable allowances for (1) the need to balance the interests of the host country against those of DoD and the U.S., and (2) the varying governmental infrastructures in the different countries?

d. How well does each strategic plan respond to the particular infectious disease surveillance challenges and the cultural dictates extant in the region in which it is to be implemented?

e. How well are the laboratories working on the other goals of GEIS (response, training and capacity building, and research) in support of their surveillance activities?

The committee will also assess:

f. How well are GEIS program goals, objectives, and activities being carried out domestically, namely, within the military health system (MHS) and the GEIS Central Hub?

## THE STUDY PROCESS

The IOM convened a committee, the Committee to Review the Department of Defense Global Emerging Infections Surveillance and Response System, at the request of GEIS management. The study began in April 2000 with a meeting, held in Washington, D.C., to familiarize the committee with GEIS. As part of that meeting, the committee received overview presentations and documentation regarding GEIS laboratory programs and was provided with the 5-year GEIS project plans developed by each of the overseas laboratories (the plans referred to in the committee's statement of task).

Thereafter, committee members made site visits to each of five DoD overseas laboratories. Between June and October 2000, teams of two to three committee members each visited Naval Medical Research Center Detachment, Peru; Naval Medical Research Unit 2, Indonesia; the Armed Forces Research Institute of Medical Sciences, Thailand; Naval Medical Research Unit 3, Egypt; and the U.S. Army Medical Research Unit, Kenya. The visits lasted approximately 1 week at each laboratory. During the site visits, committee members toured laboratory facilities, attended briefings and presentations, and met with laboratory staff and collaborators.

The scope of the study was expanded in November 2000 to include review of GEIS activities within the MHS and the Central Hub as well. As part of that review, the committee visited the Naval Health Research Center,[5] San Diego, California, and USAMRIID in Washington, D.C. It was not practical to visit all MHS sites hosting GEIS-funded projects. Instead, the committee relied heavily on written documents and summary presentations from and discussions with DoD personnel and collaborators to gain an understanding of these efforts. All told, six site visits and five committee meetings (one of which included a trip to USAMRIID) were held during the course of the study.

## APPROACHING THE TASK

As the committee learned more about GEIS, it became increasingly apparent that addressing several elements of the statement of task required careful consideration and interpretation. These are described in the following sections.

### Focus on Written Plans

The committee reviewed considerable written background information, including the 5-year operating plans for each overseas laboratory, during the course of its study. The laboratory plans, presented to the committee in April 2000, detail planned GEIS projects at overseas laboratories for fiscal years 2000 through 2004. These plans are informative, but they do not in and of themselves provide a particularly complete, current, or in-practice picture of GEIS activities at the overseas laboratories. Site visits and presentations—contractually specified elements of the study process—provided much richer information. The committee interpreted its charge as intending consideration of all information available, including, but not limited to, information contained in laboratory plan documents.

Similarly, the committee found that its charge left room for interpretation regarding how narrowly or broadly the review should be focused. It was not feasible to conduct a technical review of GEIS-supported projects (such is the level of detail presented in the laboratory plans). The duration of the study (18 months) exceeded the annual GEIS project cycle, rendering any project-specific guidance that the committee might offer

---

[5]During this trip, the committee also visited the Navy Environmental and Preventive Medicine Unit 5, and the U.S. Naval Hospital, San Diego.

potentially obsolete by the time of the study's completion. Although timely, scientific evaluation of projects is certainly valuable, the IOM committee process did not seem to provide an appropriate vehicle for this exercise. As such, although the committee considered specific projects in the course of its review, the committee focused its efforts on developing conclusions and recommendations with long-term, program-level relevance rather than on evaluating specific GEIS projects.

### Focus on Overseas Laboratories

As noted previously, the initial intent of the study was to provide a review of GEIS implementation at DoD overseas laboratories. The scope of the committee's task was later expanded to incorporate evaluation of non-overseas laboratory GEIS elements as well, specifically, GEIS activities addressed within the infrastructure of the MHS and through the GEIS Central Hub. The purpose of this task expansion was, as the committee understood it, to permit a complete review of GEIS. Although a task item was added (task f), the wording "overseas laboratory" still permeates the charge. The committee interprets the elements of its task as collectively intending review of GEIS as a whole.

### Tools for Review

GEIS is a composite program sustained through a diverse collection of activities carried out by a diverse and diffuse set of consortium members. WHO and CDC standard guidelines for the evaluation of surveillance systems (CDC, 1999, 2000; Klaucke et al., 1988; WHO, 1999a,b, 2001b) exist to guide formal reviews of national and state surveillance systems. They are not appropriate tools for direct application when reviewing GEIS activities at overseas laboratories and other DoD facilities or for use in evaluating GEIS as a whole. The committee interpreted its task as indicating that WHO and CDC guidelines may be used as reference tools but that strict adherence to WHO or CDC surveillance system review formats is not required.

The committee used WHO and CDC guidelines to direct the form and content of its site visits to the overseas laboratories. The type of descriptive information that the committee collected and the approach used to collect it particularly reflect CDC guidance (CDC, 1999, 2000). The overseas laboratory evaluations presented in this report are loosely modeled on WHO-specified surveillance system assessment domains[6] (WHO,

[6]That is, priority diseases, capacity, coordination-synergy, and laboratory assessment domains.

1999a, 2001b), which were adapted to reflect the characteristics of GEIS, the unique circumstances of the overseas laboratories, and the requirements and limitations of this review. Furthermore, members of this committee are quite familiar with CDC and WHO surveillance system evaluation procedures and were able to bring this knowledge to bear in identifying information areas to be addressed.

Similarly, the committee interprets its charge as calling for comparison of the GEIS approach to emerging infectious disease surveillance with IOM recommendations[7] and CDC strategies at the program level (rather than using GEIS activities at each laboratory as the basis of comparison). It is GEIS as a whole that has an "approach"—presented in the GEIS strategic plan (GEIS, 1998)—to emerging infectious disease surveillance. GEIS activities carried out at DoD laboratories are a part of this approach.

## THE FORMAT OF THIS REPORT

Chapters 2 through 6 of this report contain descriptions, conclusions, and recommendations regarding the implementation of GEIS at each of the five DoD overseas laboratories. Conclusions and recommendations are specific to the respective chapters. Chapter 7 of this report presents the committee's descriptions, conclusions, and recommendations regarding GEIS activities carried out within the MHS infrastructure and through the GEIS Central Hub. The committee's evaluations of these activities were conducted differently than the overseas laboratory evaluations, and the format of Chapter 7 reflects this. The recommendations and conclusions presented in Chapter 7 reflect summary committee assessments of MHS and Central Hub activities and are specific to that chapter.

Chapter 8 of this report presents summary conclusions and recommendations regarding GEIS as a whole. These are based on what the committee learned during its assessments of the respective parts of GEIS. The conclusions and recommendations presented in Chapter 8 are derived from information presented in Chapters 2 through 7 but are not repetitions of the text in those chapters.

---

[7]The committee interprets "the IOM report on emerging infectious disease" as referring specifically to the seminal 1992 publication, *Emerging Infections: Microbial Threats to Health in the United States* (IOM, 1992).

# 2

# GEIS at Naval Medical Research Center Detachment, Peru

The Naval Medical Research Center Detachment, Peru (NMRCD; formerly the Naval Medical Research Institute Detachment [NAMRID]), facility in Lima was established in 1983 through an agreement between the surgeons general of the Peruvian and U.S. Navies, with the concurrence of the U.S. Department of State and the Peruvian Ministry of Foreign Affairs. The agreement established a cooperative medical research program to study infectious diseases of interest to both parties. NMRCD is a field detachment of its parent command, the Naval Medical Research Center, Forest Glen, Maryland (GEIS, 2000g; NMRCD, 2000d).

Historically, NMRCD has focused on applied research in support of its medical mission. Its past research focus provides a strong framework for the U.S. Department of Defense (DoD) Global Emerging Infections Surveillance and Response System (GEIS) focus on surveillance and response capacity. NMRCD projects receive funding from numerous sources, including the Military Infectious Disease Research Program, the Southern Command (SOUTHCOM), and GEIS. GEIS funding for NMRCD activities totaled $950,000 in fiscal year 2000 (GEIS, 2000b) and is expected to total $1,075,000 in 2001 (GEIS, 2000c).

A subcommittee of the Institute of Medicine (IOM) Committee to Review the Department of Defense Global Emerging Infections Surveillance and Response System visited NMRCD from June 19 to 23, 2000. The subcommittee consisted of committee members Kathleen Gensheimer and Ronald St. John, accompanied by Institute of Medicine staff member Heather O'Maonaigh. A list of the people met and interviewed and the itinerary followed can be found at the end of this chapter.

## LABORATORY

NMRCD's primary laboratory facility is housed within a 33,000-square-foot laboratory and animal research unit in Lima, Peru. Within this facility is maintained a traditional scientific organizational structure consisting of bacteriology, virology, parasitology, and entomology departments. NMRCD's Lima laboratory is equipped to support medical research- and disease surveillance-related activities, activities that use approaches ranging from classical microbiology to modern molecular biology-based approaches. The laboratory animal facility is accredited by the Association for Assessment and Accreditation of Laboratory Animal Care–International. A field laboratory in Iquitos, Peru, provides an operational base site for ecological and epidemiological studies, including disease surveillance, in the Amazon basin (GEIS, 2000b; NMRCD, 2000c; Watts, 1996). The Iquitos laboratory facility is equipped primarily for specimen collection and processing.

The NMRCD laboratory facility in Lima possesses biosafety level 2 (BSL-2) and incomplete BSL-3 capacities. Specimens from fatal cases and pathogens with rapid incubation periods are sent to collaborators and supporting facilities that possess BSL-4 capabilities for analysis. Strong linkages with the Centers for Disease Control and Prevention (CDC) and the University of Texas Medical Branch, Galveston, as well as the U.S. Army Medical Research Institute for Infectious Disease, enhance NMRCD's ability to identify new or novel pathogens.

The Peruvian health authorities have accepted a paradigm shift from surveillance of laboratory-confirmed diagnoses to syndromic surveillance, which blends epidemiology with clinical findings and laboratory diagnosis, as required. Expanding laboratory diagnostic capacity is, however, a Peruvian public health priority. The Instituto Nacional de Salud (INS; Peruvian National Institutes of Health) serves as the national reference laboratory for Peru. It is currently supporting the decentralization of laboratory capacity to 14 of Peru's 34 health regions. In addition, the INS is constructing a BSL-2 laboratory in Iquitos and a BSL-2 and BSL-3 facility in Lima. Currently, the largest-capacity laboratory maintained by the INS operates at BSL-2 and is located in Lima. NMRCD uses its laboratory capacity to support Peruvian infectious disease surveillance efforts by augmenting regional laboratory supplies and providing specimen-processing assistance when requested. The INS has identified as priority areas regional laboratory capacity in diarrheal disease diagnosis, serological testing, and quality assurance of antibiotic resistance testing. These priority areas are largely compatible with GEIS project areas, and the INS welcomes GEIS-supported surveillance projects.

### Conclusions

Laboratory capacity at current BSL levels, augmented by collaborating laboratory networks, is sufficient to support GEIS. The NMRCD laboratory facility in Lima provides a good example of close collaboration between U.S. and national laboratories. Support for such a collaboration is one of the objectives of GEIS (GEIS, 1998).

## STAFFING

At the time of the IOM subcommittee's visit, NMRCD staff included six professional, uniformed services personnel[1]: the officer in charge (a Navy commander, physician-epidemiologist); the head of the Bacteriology Department, who also serves as the manager of GEIS (a Navy captain, microbiologist); a scientist assigned from the CDC (a Public Health Service captain, physician-epidemiologist); the head of the Virology Department (a Navy lieutenant commander, epidemiologist-physician); the head of the Entomology Department; and a scientific director, based in Washington, D.C. An Army physician-investigator was added to the NMRCD staff shortly after the subcommittee's visit. Three more professional personnel are to be added to the NMRCD staff in the coming year, as are an administrative officer, a biomedical repair technician, and a veterinary technician.

In addition, NMRCD employs a staff of foreign service nationals (FSNs), including 22 administrative support and 19 research personnel. FSN staff include laboratory technicians, a veterinarian, and contract personnel with expertise in the areas of departmental focus. Dedicated, contracted field personnel manage NMRCD field operations on a full-time basis. No full-time employee works exclusively on GEIS projects. All department heads have significant involvement in programs other than GEIS.

### Conclusions

The NMRCD hosts a dedicated, skilled scientific team that attempts to fulfill GEIS objectives. At present, the program is efficiently run under the direction of its program manager, but because his responsibilities also

[1]The subcommittee's visit took place at a time of transition in NMRCD personnel. Both a new officer in charge and a new Entomology Department head were installed at NMRCD as of June 2000. Also, as of August 1, 2000, an Army physician-investigator was assigned to NMRCD.

include directing the Bacteriology Department, continued coordination of GEIS may be difficult. The project is given strong support from the NMRCD officer in charge (transitioning out at the time of the subcommittee visit), who has worked diligently to lay a strong foundation to secure the success of the GEIS mission.

Currently, the CDC epidemiologist who is assigned to NMRCD and who heads GEIS's antimalarial drug resistance projects offers some needed support in public health and applied epidemiology. However, the CDC epidemiologist is clearly occupied with directing the various components of the malaria studies and is not available to provide the overall epidemiological support that GEIS requires.

The subcommittee was impressed with the high level of staff (DoD and contract personnel) commitment to and enthusiasm for GEIS projects. Staff relationships appeared to be supportive and mutually reinforcing. However, duty assignments to NMRCD frequently last only one rotation (generally 2 to 4 years), and the costs of employee turnover are high. Longer terms of service (more than one rotation) contribute to the formation and enhancement of working relationships and are of particular importance given the emphasis of GEIS on collaborative activities. NMRCD connections with agencies and organizations central to Peru's political and public health infrastructures are jeopardized when staff changes occur, potentially affecting GEIS activities. Increased hiring and assignment of U.S. civilian and FSN scientists can help to ameliorate this issue.

## TECHNOLOGY AND INFORMATION MANAGEMENT

Within NMRCD's Lima laboratory, communications systems provide e-mail, Internet, fax, and telephone access. An on-site data center supplies computer systems support, as well as data entry and analysis services and surveillance data reporting, as needed. At the Iquitos field site, access to e-mail, fax, telephone, and photocopying capabilities are available. Within the NMRCD laboratory, frozen specimen archives are maintained, but they are not cataloged electronically. A version of the Laboratory Information Tracking System Plus software, developed by the CDC, is to be modified and used to catalog this information once a useable version of this application is available.

### Conclusions

A tour of the NMRCD facility and its field site in Iquitos impressed the subcommittee members with the sophistication of the technology available. Computer and communications technologies (access to the World Wide Web, e-mail, library facilities, and an office computer network) appeared to be sufficient to support GEIS. The planned addition of an electronic specimen-cataloging system is an important effort that coincides with GEIS's goals (GEIS, 1998).

## SURVEILLANCE[2]

The GEIS focus on surveillance and response capacity was added in fiscal year 1997 to the existing NMRCD operating structure, which was historically dedicated to laboratory-based medical research. At NMRCD GEIS is conceptually organized around five pillars, four of which were defined by the GEIS Central Hub and one of which (entomological surveillance) was added by NMRCD. These pillars are (NMRCD, 2000a,c)

- drug-resistant malaria surveillance,
- influenza surveillance,
- surveillance for drug-resistant enteric pathogens,
- acute febrile illness (AFI) surveillance, and
- entomological surveillance (specifically, insect vectors of the malaria parasite and arboviruses).

GEIS-related pillars are integrated across all four NMRCD departments, with department heads using existing personnel to support the work of GEIS. Within each pillar, NMRCD has developed several specific projects. In fiscal year 1999, NMRCD GEIS-funded projects involved sentinel surveillance for influenza, antibiotic-resistant enteric infections, and antimalarial drug resistance (GEIS, 1999a).

NMRCD is essentially rebuilding programs that faltered during the 1990–1995 period of terrorism in Peru. Most GEIS projects are in their infancies; others are still waiting to begin. Initially, a great deal of effort was spent to prepare for GEIS implementation and integration with national and other partners. Most GEIS projects are in their first year of full funding. Projects funded in fiscal years 2000 to 2004 include continued studies of drug-resistant malaria, surveillance for influenza and drug-resistant enteric bacteria, as well as projects addressing acute febrile illness and entomological surveillance activities.

### *Drug-Resistant Malaria Surveillance*

Antimalarial drug resistance monitoring is to be conducted during fiscal year 2000–2001 at sites in Peru, Surinam, Bolivia, and Ecuador.

[2]The summaries in this section reflect project planning at the time of the subcommittee site visit in June 2000. At that time, many projects were in their planning stage or had recently begun.

Project collaborators include the Walter Reed Army Institute of Research, the Naval Medical Research Center, the CDC, and the University of Toronto, as well as the Pan American Health Organization, the INS, the Peruvian Navy, and ministries of health. Clinical and parasitological failures of antimalarial drug therapy will be studied in patients with *Plasmodium falciparum* or *Plasmodium vivax* infections. In vivo testing of approximately 50 specimens per surveillance site will be conducted each year, with in vitro testing conducted where logistically possible. Training of Ministry of Health personnel will be undertaken as part of this work. The long-term goal of this project is the transfer of a sustainable antimalarial drug resistance program to host country public health authorities (NMRCD, 2000a,b).

*Influenza Surveillance*

Specimens containing influenza virus are to be collected at U.S. embassy health units, as well as surveillance sites, and forwarded to the DoD Laboratory-Based Influenza Surveillance Program at Brooks Air Force Base in San Antonio, Texas, for virus isolation and characterization. Basic demographic information will be collected at the time of specimen collection. Approximately 40 samples are to be collected per site per year. Influenza surveillance sites have already been established in Argentina, Ecuador, and Peru. Additional sites are planned in Chile, Bolivia, and Ecuador. Secondary goals of this project include the training of locals and capacity building (NMRCD, 2000a,b).

*Surveillance for Enteric Pathogens*

NMRCD has sporadically collected enteric bacterial isolates for several years, but now, under the auspices of GEIS, plans for a more systematic surveillance effort are in place. Surveillance sites have been established in Bolivia, and there are plans to include sites in Peru and Ecuador as well. No plan to collect specimens from the U.S. embassy population was noted. The number of antibiotics used in resistance screening will be increased from 7 to 13. Samples (25 from each site) will be collected from surveillance sites during four peak periods of diarrheal occurrence each year (NMRCD, 2000a,b).

*Acute Febrile Illness Surveillance*

Specimens from patients presenting with undifferentiated fevers will be collected from sites in Peru and a site in Bolivia, with plans to add a surveillance site in Ecuador at a later date. Samples are to be collected from 250 individuals from each site during the first year of the study (calendar year 2000). Viral isolations will be performed with acute-phase serum specimens. Serologies will be performed with convalescent-phase serum specimens. Patients will be characterized as presenting with undifferentiated febrile syndrome, undifferentiated febrile syndrome with rash, hemorrhagic fever syndrome, febrile icteric syndrome, and acute respiratory syndrome. This study will be linked with other GEIS efforts, such as entomological, influenza, and antimalarial drug resistance surveillance activities. Improvements in regional laboratory capacity and the training of locals are additional benefits of this work. Local collaborators will be encouraged to make project data available to in-country surveillance networks, but NMRCD will not report the data directly (NMRCD, 2000a,b).

### *Entomological Surveillance Activities*

Arthropod vector surveillance is to be conducted at Puerto Almendras, a site near Iquitos, in the Amazon, and at a site near Tarapoto, in the foothills of the Andes. Mosquitoes will be collected by a variety of methods. Surveillance events being monitored are the introduction of new mosquito species, changes in the distribution of previously known species, the identification of previously unrecognized vectors, characterization of the behaviors of important vectors, and the identification of arboviruses. Surveillance will be carried out at health clinics proximate to the mosquito surveillance sites to determine if viruses detected in the mosquito populations are appearing in humans (NMRCD, 2000a,b).

### *Considerations*

NMRCD GEIS projects are designed to investigate the descriptive epidemiology of selected diseases in sentinel sites. AFI, enteric pathogens, and influenza projects use sentinel sites to access populations that are strategically located in all three of Peru's ecological zones, namely, the coastal desert area, the lower highlands and northern coast, and the tropical eastern area. Sentinel sites have also been developed in neighboring Bolivia and Ecuador. Surveillance is limited to patients seeking care from public health care facilities. Thus, the projects sample only a portion of the Peruvian population in distinct ecological zones. For example, the National Social Security System, which provides clinical care for 25 percent of the Peruvian population, remains outside the scope of GEIS surveillance activities. Sampling from sentinel sites has some inherent limitations, including potential biases associated with site selection, health care-seeking behavior, clinical decisions to obtain laboratory samples, and the effects of previous self-medication. Data obtained from sentinel surveillance systems may not be generalizable to the entire population of interest. Sentinel surveillance is, however, a reasonable approach for a supplemental surveillance activity such as GEIS.

To understand NMRCD's role in infectious disease surveillance in Peru, it is important to consider the existing surveillance systems in the host country with which GEIS should interact. The Peruvian Ministry of Health, in collaboration with the U.S. Agency for International Development (USAID), has dedicated many resources to strengthening Peru's national computerized surveillance system. In response to national priorities, USAID developed the Addressing Threats of Emerging and Re-Emerging Infectious Diseases (VIGIA) project in late 1997. This project is funded at $24 million ($18 million from USAID funds and $6 million from the Peruvian government) over a period of approximately 6 years (through September 30, 2004) (USAID and U.S. Embassy, Lima, Peru, 2000).

The system is designed to build local capacity for data collection, data analysis, and response, including reporting and local investigation of epidemics. It is based on electronic linking of approximately 6,000 local health districts to the central Oficina General de Epidemiologia (OGE; Office of Epidemiology, Peruvian Ministry of Health) through the 34 health regions in Peru. Each district reports cases of notifiable infectious diseases to a health region on a weekly basis. Each region has a health situation room where weekly data are tabulated in graphic format and displayed on the walls. The rate of compliance with weekly reporting was stated to be approximately 90 percent. Each health region is linked to OGE by Internet television for visual conferences and rapid reporting and discussion of unusual situations. In many respects, the communications technology possessed by OGE is superior to the communications technology available at NMRCD.

Since 1998, to staff this electronic system, Peru has provided basic training in epidemiology for approximately 900 people for district-level work. Three hundred people received more advanced training in epidemiology for region-level work, whereas 90 people received even more advanced training for work at the national level. In addition, 30 people received full training in epidemiology at the master's level. This training program is operated under the aegis of the Peruvian Field Epidemiology Training Program, but it lacks a field training component and is considered to be weak.

The current surveillance system generates local epidemiological bulletins and early warnings and alerts. Although the USAID investment is creating an impressive surveillance infrastructure for the rapid reporting of the incidence and prevalence of 14 legally notifiable infectious diseases, several observers noted that there is still room for greater analysis of the available data and for the subsequent use of the resulting information to formulate national health policy and to generate public health action. It was noted, for example, that although the system generates a large amount of information of variable quality (not all data are coherent and internally consistent), the information generated is sufficient for a rough analysis of the local epidemiological profile and general infectious disease trends, but many of the data do not appear to be analyzed and converted into appropriate and timely public health action.[3]

The objective of OGE is to produce local data for local analysis and local decision making. During the visit to the regional health office in Iquitos, it was not apparent how well this process was working. There also appeared to be a lack of understanding regarding the goals of GEIS. When asked what GEIS could contribute at the regional level, the response from the OGE medical director was that GEIS could (1) conduct studies of hepatitis B and hepatitis delta viruses, (2) study the virology of diarrheal diseases, (3) provide more equipment for the regional laboratory, and (4) continue facilitating specimen transportation to Lima. These region-level wants do not seem to fall clearly within the mission of GEIS or the scope of its current project areas. At the OGE central level, the information and support contributed by GEIS were recognized and valued.

## Conclusions

NMRCD's laboratory capacity helps support the Peruvian national surveillance system by reinforcing INS laboratory capacity. Additionally, GEIS at NMRCD can serve a data quality assurance function by providing data from its studies to the INS and OGE. At present, the exchange of data and other information between NMRCD and its partners is project dependent and intermittent. NMRCD GEIS contributions to Peruvian surveillance efforts would be bolstered by the more systematic and timely exchange of information. GEIS also contributes to infectious disease surveillance in Peru through training and capacity building. It is primarily through laboratory capacity building and support and through other indirect means such as training that NMRCD GEIS is of benefit to Peru's infectious disease surveillance system.

With the exception of the influenza surveillance pillar, GEIS project areas and Peruvian national epidemiological priorities are compatible. Malaria parasite antimalarial drug resistance, enteric pathogen antimicrobial drug resistance, and undiagnosed fevers (especially those due to arboviruses, such as dengue virus) are all national health concerns.

---

[3]The subcommittee did not have time to verify the validity of the large amount of data being generated or to explore how these data were being used to influence national health policies.

GEIS efforts to examine drug-resistant malaria and drug-resistant enteric disease are of undeniable importance and are well matched with Peruvian health objectives; however, the subcommittee questions the public health value of the entomological surveillance studies. Much of this entomological surveillance work appears to be a virus hunt, about which the subcommittee has mixed feelings. Certainly, one cannot argue against the research-related importance of identifying new viruses; however, the public health relevance of the information that these studies will generate is questionable. When a new virus is identified in mosquito populations, such information may not be relevant for public health policy. This work would result in greater public health contributions if targeted to populated areas of high viral disease endemicity.

The subcommittee recognizes the value of influenza surveillance in South America. Such information is useful to the World Health Organization's (WHO's) influenza surveillance system (FLUNET). At the Peruvian national level, where little influenza vaccine is used, the usefulness of such information is questionable. However, NMRCD GEIS influenza surveillance projects are low cost as a result of ties with the DoD Laboratory-Based Influenza Surveillance Program, and they are of use to the global community. For example, specimens sent by NMRCD to the DoD Laboratory-Based Influenza Surveillance Program in April 1999 identified the presence of the influenza strain A/New Caledonia/20/99 in the Americas and influenced the WHO recommendation to include this strain in the 2000 Southern Hemisphere and the 2000–2001 Northern Hemisphere vaccines (Gaydos, 2001d; GEIS, 2000b; Kelley, 2000b).

The head of the Department of Virology, who is the director of the AFI studies, has developed a very comprehensive and reasonable network of sentinel study sites. He approximates that 20 percent of the febrile illnesses in Peru are attributable to the malaria parasites and that another 20 percent are attributable to arboviruses. An important question—one that GEIS AFI studies seek to address—is, What contributes to the remaining 60 percent of these syndromes? The study sites that have been established to address this question will be very helpful in addressing febrile illness-related morbidity in Peru.

Despite the value of current GEIS project areas, many potentially important surveillance activities are left unaddressed. The subcommittee repeatedly heard concerns about respiratory disease syndromes and acute pneumonias; however, GEIS projects do not include these diseases. Multidrug-resistant (MDR) tuberculosis (MDR-TB) is another disease entity that looms as a public health threat on a global basis. Although MDR-TB does not pose a direct threat to military security, it certainly poses a direct threat to the developing world, and if it is not brought under control, it will continue to pose a threat to U.S. citizens. To the extent that military personnel deployed overseas become infected with MDR *Mycobacterium tuberculosis*, the risk to the U.S. civilian population is increased. The subcommittee questions how best to balance GEIS interests to evaluate not only those disease entities that may pose a direct threat to the U.S. military but also to integrate such surveillance and public health efforts with the needs of the host country, such as hepatitis B and hepatitis delta viruses.[4]

The subcommittee also questions whether the current annual review and funding process allows sufficient time for surveillance project maturation and planning between reviews. Annual review appears to rush the proposal preparation process and can culminate in the making of decisions about the merits of projects on the basis of incomplete information.

## RESPONSE CAPACITY

NMRCD staff have participated in several investigations of epidemics. The processes leading to a response to an epidemic and the methods of epidemic response are described as varied. Response efforts are led by the Ministry of Health and, as needed, the involvement of NMRCD and other partners (e.g., the WHO and the CDC) is sought.

As GEIS project data accumulate, ongoing epidemiological analyses of these data may be used to identify unusual events and possible epidemics for rapid reporting to OGE. Data linkages to OGE may facilitate ongoing monitoring of results from studies such as the AFI surveillance project.

### Conclusions

At NMRCD, GEIS possesses resources (e.g., laboratory capacity, staff expertise, and collaborative relationships) that can be and that have been put to use in response to warnings of epidemics in Peru and the region. GEIS can foster NMRCD involvement in response efforts by supporting the prompt reporting of project data to OGE and by strengthening the ties between NMRCD and the Peruvian public health network.

## COLLABORATIONS

Steps have been taken to integrate GEIS with current, ongoing activities at the INS, OGE, and the Universidad Peruana Cayetano de Heredia—

[4]Also of potential public health interest: only 50 to 60 percent of the deaths in Peru are registered, potentially masking emerging infectious disease threats. Sentinel surveillance of deaths in the 15- to 49-year-old age group may uncover deaths due to unrecognized infectious causes (PAHO, 1998, pp. 415–421).

key components of Peru's public health infrastructure. In-country relationships are largely person based rather than position based, and partnerships have benefited from staffing and programmatic changes at NMRCD and other agencies in recent years. GEIS staff seemed to be very well known and respected by the local and regional health officials.

Collaborative relationships between organizations and agencies with public health interests in Peru (including agencies of the Peruvian government, the U.S. government, and international organizations) are quite complex. Of interest, the subcommittee heard various accounts of which disease entities posed public health challenges. Close collaborations are essential in making such determinations. The observed lack of concurrence suggests that the relationships observed could be more robust.

Orientation slides provided to the subcommittee by OGE made no mention of GEIS or NMRCD, although other relationships were specified. VIGIA staff noted that NMRCD was helpful in maintaining relationships with U.S. laboratories; that NMRCD aided in the discovery of new viruses and bacteria; that NMRCD provided technical backup for the INS, especially in the area of quality assurance; that NMRCD assisted with technology transfer and laboratory training; and that NMRCD participated in and supported investigations of epidemics. VIGIA staff did not note a role for GEIS in the Peruvian surveillance system per se, despite similarities between the surveillance goals of VIGIA and GEIS.

NMRCD also serves an important training role. NMRCD has offered at-the-bench laboratory training for a variety of national (Ryan, 2000) and international personnel. Medical students, residents, and visiting faculty, both national and international, have benefited from time spent at NMRCD in various training modes.

## Conclusions

NMRCD staff currently involved with GEIS understand the need to establish collaborative and collegial networks with the Peruvian scientific and public health communities, and their efforts to do so are slowly producing positive results. In these regards, special credit needs to be given to the energy and vitality that FSN staff members bring to the program. Of note, the FSN contractor serving as the GEIS assistant manager understands the dynamics of the Peruvian scientific and governmental public health communities. She has worked to establish and maintain relationships that will be vital to the success and integration of the work of GEIS into the Peruvian public health infrastructure. In addition, the FSN manager of the Iquitos field site has an understanding of the NMRCD mission, as a result of her years of working in the Lima laboratory before transferring to Iquitos. Her interaction with the local population is critical to the success of the studies implemented in this Amazon field station. This staff support is instrumental in surmounting the many challenges posed by the complex organizational relationships that exist in Peru.

To facilitate productive partnerships, it is useful for GEIS staff to have, at a minimum, a working conversational level of proficiency in Spanish. Attempts must be made to interact with Peruvian officials in their native language. That effort is not only appreciated but also works to assimilate staff into the local culture, an understanding of which promotes optimal working relationships.

If GEIS is to be successful, NMRCD must continue to work through the complex set of relationships that exist within Peru and continue its work with other in-country organizations and agencies on a continual and productive basis. Closer collaboration, more coordination, and better communication are goals toward which all in-country parties need to strive. The subcommittee noted, for example, that there appears to be weak integration of GEIS and NMRCD capacity with the USAID-VIGIA project, despite NMRCD's efforts to engage USAID as a partner. The subcommittee recognizes that, in many cases, improvements in relationships between organizations must follow improvements in coordination and communication within the organizations themselves.

GEIS at NMRCD might, for example, benefit from clearer communication and closer coordination with the GEIS Central Hub. For example, INS staff noted that the recent introduction of Public Health Laboratory Information System (PHLIS) software into the INS could have been better coordinated between the GEIS Central Hub and NMRCD GEIS staff. Benefits may also be obtained by encouraging working relationships between the GEIS overseas laboratories. For instance, it may be useful to have the coordinators for all GEIS projects on AFI in all DoD laboratories develop criteria for definitions of cases for syndromic surveillance instead of having each site struggle with such criteria on its own.

The review team heard several comments regarding the forms of support that NMRCD should be offering to in-country programs. Most of the comments concerned provision of more laboratory support (e.g., offering quality assurance programs for laboratories) and provision of laboratory equipment and reagents. The boundaries of GEIS are difficult to define, as GEIS responsibilities to the host country are not always clear. Clarification of this point would be useful to GEIS and to its in-country partners.

NMRCD has worked to promote an extensive training role in the Peruvian medical community and also provides training for DoD personnel and other students. Such efforts can be expanded through GEIS. However, training is a time-consuming activity, especially in the absence of a planned, formal training program with a set of organized courses to meet needs for specific skill sets. The subcommittee noted the absence of a training officer to coordinate formal training programs in collaboration with Peruvian nationals.

## RECOMMENDATIONS

• GEIS activities at NMRCD are critical to GEIS as a whole. The committee encourages the DoD to plan for GEIS activities at NMRCD on a long-term basis. NMRCD provides a unique resource for research and for public health missions. Demand for and support of these missions should be balanced so that neither is jeopardized.

**Recommendation: DoD commitment to GEIS at NMRCD should be long term.**

• It is important that unmet GEIS staffing needs be addressed. New positions should be created, as needed, to meet these needs.

**Recommendation: Full-time staff members should be assigned to NMRCD to meet staffing needs in the following areas:**

**GEIS program management. The GEIS program manager should not have simultaneous responsibility for departmental management and administering overall NMRCD GEIS activities. The GEIS program manager should be full-time and on-site, and should possess, at a minimum, applied epidemiology and public health experience.**

**Support of training activities. The coordination of training activities is an important but time-intensive GEIS task. This task should not be consigned to NMRCD department heads as a secondary responsibility.**

**Epidemiology. Additional epidemiological support (including, but not necessarily limited to, a dedicated GEIS program manager) should be provided to help facilitate public health-oriented data analysis and study design and to provide a permanent link between NMRCD and the OGE national surveillance system, as well as other public health partners.**

**Administrative support. Extensive administrative requirements can impede the work of a scientific staff that is already stretched thin. Additional administrative (nonclerical) support should be provided so that NMRCD scientists can devote their talents to GEIS studies under way.**

• Partnerships benefit from knowledge of the native language by senior staff. Partnerships are of increased importance to NMRCD now that its research mission has been expanded to include GEIS activities, which necessitate more interaction with partner agencies. Staff familiarity and comfort with the local language can also improve personnel retention.

**Recommendation: NMRCD senior staff who are actively involved in GEIS projects should be conversant in the dominant language of**

**the host country or should pursue, with the support of GEIS, language training, and should seek to become conversant to the extent possible.**

• Training local personnel in laboratory technology and providing an opportunity for DoD personnel and students to receive research training are important ways in which GEIS is and can increasingly be of benefit to Peru and the DoD. Consolidating and coordinating NMRCD's various training activities under the aegis of GEIS may make training activities more efficient, productive, and visible.

**Recommendation: DoD and Peruvian training needs should be assessed formally, and the development of a structured NMRCD-hosted training program should be considered.**

• The reporting of data to Peruvian authorities should be timely and systematic and needs to be targeted toward achieving public health action.

**Recommendation: As GEIS project data are accumulated, they should be better used to supplement the OGE national surveillance system, provide early warnings of epidemics, and help guide public health responses.**

• NMRCD has established connections with the political and public health infrastructures in Peru and understands the subtleties of how to operate effectively in country. NMRCD should continue to strengthen and expand these connections. In particular, improved coordination between members of the U.S. team in country should be pursued. For example, NMRCD should continue to seek to be more involved in the ongoing planning and implementation of the USAID-VIGIA project. To these ends, assistance from the regional unified combatant command (SOUTHCOM) and the U.S. ambassador should be sought, as needed.

**Recommendation: NMRCD should take continued steps to maintain and enhance the multiple national and international partnerships that are necessary to fulfill the GEIS mission and build national capacity in Peru.**

• The subcommittee recognizes that the GEIS pillar disease areas are important ones and that defining these targets helps to provide some standardization of GEIS activities across sites, but the pillar structure should be flexible enough to permit, on a case-by-case basis, local infectious diseases that are of global concern (e.g., tuberculosis) to be addressed as high priorities through GEIS. This serves to take full advantage of the epidemiological setting of the facility, builds national health defenses in the host country, and can be of long-term benefit to the health of many populations, including U.S. military personnel and civilians.

**Recommendation: Consideration should be given to refining the focus of GEIS at NMRCD to better enable diseases outside of the pillar areas to be addressed.**

• The current annual approval process does not allow optimal time for NMRCD project planning or maturation. Furthermore, it is important that the GEIS Central Hub review and approval process for GEIS projects provides NMRCD with follow-up guidance regarding project progress in a consistent and timely manner (see also Chapter 7).

**Recommendation: Consideration should be given to revising the current GEIS project application and review process.**

## PEOPLE MET AND INTERVIEWED

### *NMRCD Staff*

LCDR Kevin Russell, head, Department of Virology
CAPT Trenton Ruebush, Public Health Service/CDC, Malaria Drug Resistance
CAPT Stephen Walz, head, Department of Microbiology, and head, GEIS Program
Dr. Monica Negrete, GEIS assistant manager
Dr. Douglas Watts, scientific director
CDR Trueman Sharp, officer in charge at the time of the subcommittee visit
CDR (Select) James Burans, replacing CDR Sharp as officer in charge
Carla Block, manager, Iquitos Field Site
Jorge Cervantes, assistant, Iquitos Field Site

### *NMRCD Associates*

Ambassador John Hamilton, United States
COL Gilbert R. Perez, USA, Special Forces, Chief, MAAG-Peru
Dr. O. Jaime Chang, coordinator, VIGIA project
Dr. Eduardo Falconi Rosadio, Instituto Nacional de Salud
Dr. Luis Seminario Carrasco, asesor en salud, Oficina De Salud, Nutricion y Poblacion, USAID
Dr. Percy Minaya Leon, director, General Office of Epidemiology
Dr. Marie Andree Diouf, representative in Peru, PAHO
Dr. Ruben Figuero, epidemiologist, PAHO

Dr. Carlos Calampa, director, Regional Health Department, Loreto Region
Dr. Ciro Maguina, director adjunto, Universidad Cayetano de Heredia

## ITINERARY

*Monday, June 19*

0715 Depart hotel for U.S. Embassy
0800 Meeting with COL Gil Perez, chief of the Military Assistance and Advisory Group and SOUTHCOM representative in Peru
0830 Meeting with Ambassador John Hamilton
0915 Depart for NMRCD
1000 Welcome and overview of NMRCD (CDR Sharp)
1045 Tour of NMRCD
1115 Overview of NMRCD GEIS (CAPT Walz)
1200 Lunch
1330 Presentations and meetings with individual NMRCD GEIS staff
1700 Depart for hotel

*Tuesday, June 20*

0730 Depart hotel
0815 Meeting with Dr. Falconi and other staff at Instituto Nacional de Salud (Peruvian National Institutes of Health)
1000 Meeting with staff of Oficina General de Epidemiologia (General Office of Epidemiology)
1130 Return to NMRCD and Lunch
1600 Flight to Iquitos
1700 Arrive Iquitos
1830 Visit NMRCD laboratory/house

*Wednesday, June 21*

0730 Visit Laboratorio Referencial Loreto
0900 Appointment with Dr. Carlos Calampa, Director, Loreto Regional Health Department
1000 Hospital de Apoyo de Iquitos
1100 Centro de Salud San Juan
1200 Lunch
1530 Leave for airport
1700 Return flight to Lima

*Thursday, June 22*

0800 Depart hotel
0830 Meeting with USAID VIGIA staff at USAID
1000 Meeting with Pan American Health Organization representative
1200 Return to NMRCD for lunch
1330 Follow-up discussions with NMRCD staff
1700 Return to hotel

*Friday, June 23*

0815 Depart hotel
0900 Meet with staff, Universidad Peruana Cayetano de Heredia
1230 Return to hotel for discussion, drafting of preliminary assessment, and assignment of writing tasks

# 3

# GEIS at Naval Medical Research Unit 2, Indonesia

Naval Medical Research Unit 2 (NAMRU-2) was established in Guam during World War II. In the years following the war, NAMRU-2 was relocated, first to Taiwan and then to the Philippines. In 1970, a NAMRU-2 detachment began operating in Jakarta, Indonesia (GEIS, 2000e). Negotiations between the U.S. Navy, the U.S. Department of State, and the government of Indonesia resulted in the transfer of the NAMRU-2 parent command from the Philippines to Jakarta in 1990 (GEIS, 2000e). The initial agreement with the Indonesian Ministry of Health (MoH) establishing NAMRU-2 command in Indonesia has recently expired, and negotiations are under way to establish a new agreement directly between the two governments. NAMRU-2 is facing some uncertainty because of political unrest in Indonesia as the country enters a period of transition from extensive autocratic rule to a democratic society.

NAMRU-2 is a subordinate command of the Naval Medical Research Center, Forest Glen, Maryland (GEIS, 2000e). NAMRU-2 is distinguished by its extremely close working relationships with Indonesian public health institutions. Projects are jointly developed and implemented with Indonesian public health officials.

Historically, NAMRU-2 has focused on applied research in support of its medical mission. Its past research focus provides a strong framework for the new focus of the U.S. Department of Defense (DoD) Global Emerging Infections Surveillance and Response System (GEIS) on surveillance and response capacity. NAMRU-2 projects receive funding from numerous sources including the Military Infectious Disease Research Program (MIDRP), GEIS, Pacific Command (PACOM), and the Navy Bureau of Medicine for administrative support, including housing and force protection. In addition, NAMRU-2 receives funding from companies like Abbott Laboratories and SmithKline for support of collaborative projects. Fiscal year 2001 GEIS funding is expected to total $1,075,000 (GEIS, 2000c).

A subcommittee of the Institute of Medicine (IOM) Committee to Review the Department of Defense Global Emerging Infections Surveillance and Response System visited NAMRU-2 from October 2 to 5, 2000. The subcommittee also visited a newly developed extension facility in Phnom Penh, Cambodia, that NAMRU-2 operates jointly with the Armed Forces Research Institute of Medical Sciences (AFRIMS), Bangkok, Thailand, on October 6 and 7, 2000. The IOM subcommittee consisted of committee members Ruth Berkelman and Ronald St. John. A list of the people met and interviewed and the itinerary followed can be found at the end of this chapter.

## LABORATORY

NAMRU-2 houses an extensive laboratory facility within a 62,000-square-foot laboratory, office, and storage space in Jakarta, Indonesia (GEIS, 2000e). The NAMRU-2 facility is collocated with the Directorate General of Communicable Disease Control and Environmental Health (a part of the MoH, hereafter referred to as "Indonesian CDC") and the Litbangkes (Indonesian National Institute of Health Research and Development, part of the Indonesian Ministry of Health). Litbangkes allocates free space on the entire third floor of its building for NAMRU-2 laboratories. NAMRU-2 also occupies a large warehouse nearby that houses additional laboratories, materials and supplies, and administrative offices. The Association for the Assessment and Accreditation of Laboratory Animal Care–International accredits NAMRU-2 laboratory animal facilities (GEIS, 2000e).

NAMRU-2's Jakarta laboratory is equipped to support medical research- and disease surveillance-related activities, activities that use approaches ranging from classical microbiology to modern molecular biology-based approaches. Within this facility, a conventional scientific organizational structure consisting of bacteriology, virology, parasitology, and entomology departments is maintained along with a recently added emerging infectious disease component. The NAMRU-2 laboratory facility in Jakarta possesses a biosafety level 2 (BSL-2) capacity and a nearly complete BSL-3 capacity. Specimens from fatal cases and pathogens with rapid incubation periods are sent to collaborators and supporting facilities that possess BSL-4 capabilities for analysis.

NAMRU-2 is establishing a subsidiary laboratory in Phnom Penh, Cambodia, to provide an operational base site to support disease surveillance and epidemiological activities. The Cambodian National Institute of

Public Health donated space for this laboratory and secured access to hospital sentinel facilities. The laboratory facility is undergoing construction and modification. This laboratory possesses a serology capacity only, but in the near future it will operate at a BSL-2 level for bacteriology. No BSL-3 level is planned. The laboratory is directed by a U.S. Centers for Disease Control and Prevention (U.S. CDC) staff person supported by NAMRU-2 through an interagency personnel agreement.

NAMRU-2 has numerous other collaborating surveillance sites throughout Indonesia and Indochina. NAMRU-2 collaborates with the National Center of Laboratory and Epidemiology and the Pasteur Institute in Vientiane, Laos, and Ho Chi Minh City, Vietnam, respectively. These associations are with host-national partners generally charged with research and surveillance activities for their respective countries. NAMRU-2 has established relationships with hospitals in Vietnam through the Pasteur Institute and via key government and public health officials who serve as collaborators and liaisons. Satellite laboratories in Lumprapang and Champassak in Laos are located in hospital compounds.

In Indonesia, a NAMRU-2 satellite laboratory facility in Jayapura (Irian Jaya) is adjacent to a hospital complex but occupies a distinct compound. NAMRU-2 personnel staff this laboratory. Additional laboratories in Medan, Bali, Jakarta, Batam, and Padang are located in network hospitals. In Pontianak and Makassar, NAMRU-2 has a presence at the provincial laboratories. Collaborative relationships have been established with numerous hospitals to collect laboratory data on diarrheal diseases (those caused by *Shigella*, *Campylobacter*, enterotoxigenic *Escherichia coli*, etc.). NAMRU-2 provides training and limited equipment and supplies to these laboratories, as well as a quality control program, and in return, it is provided with data.

The Indonesian national strategy for building a network of public health laboratories recognizes the need for a central public health reference laboratory. Laboratory services at the provincial and district levels—where capacities are variable and often rudimentary—and hospital-based laboratories fall under separate directorates in the MoH. Expansion of the laboratory diagnostic capacity in local areas is a public health priority in Indonesia. A new policy of expansion and decentralization will affect the national laboratory capacity. A planned central public health laboratory within the Indonesian CDC would serve to establish national norms, guidelines, and standards and would provide basic skills training for workers in the decentralized laboratory network. During an interview with the subcommittee team, Dr. Umar F. Achmadi, director general of the Indonesian CDC, reported that NAMRU-2 is expected to contribute to the development of this central laboratory—by assisting with standards development and staff training, for instance. NAMRU-2 uses its laboratory capacity to support Indonesian infectious disease diagnostic efforts by providing reference testing services and supporting special epidemic investigations when requested.

Strong linkages exist between NAMRU-2 and the Naval Medical Research Center, AFRIMS, the Walter Reed Army Institute of Research, and the U.S. Army Medical Research Institute for Infectious Disease. NAMRU-2 also collaborates with the U.S. CDC.

### Conclusions

Laboratory capacity in Jakarta is sufficient to support current GEIS activities in Indonesia. Construction and modification of facilities will provide sufficient space for the expansion of GEIS activities in Cambodia. Joint collaboration between the AFRIMS and NAMRU-2 will enhance the laboratory capacities for GEIS in Cambodia. Indonesian expectations of NAMRU-2 support for development of a central laboratory, including standards development and staff training, will challenge NAMRU-2 staff and will represent an added operational burden.

## STAFFING

At the time of the IOM subcommittee's visit, NAMRU-2 staff included 23 U.S. military personnel, including 14 scientists. In addition, NAMRU-2 employs a staff of more than 100 foreign service nationals (FSNs). FSN staff include laboratory technicians and contract support personnel with expertise in the areas of management and administration. Dedicated, contracted field personnel manage NAMRU-2 field operations on a full-time basis. All department heads have significant involvement in programs other than GEIS, including MIDRP projects. Within NAMRU-2, a small, dedicated Emerging Disease Program collaborates extensively with other NAMRU-2 programs and is highly dependent on them.

NAMRU-2 has recognized the advantage of having additional epidemiological expertise to support GEIS and has requested that additional U.S. CDC personnel be assigned to enhance NAMRU-2's capacity in epidemiological science.

### Conclusions

NAMRU-2 supports a dedicated, skilled scientific team that effectively fulfills the objectives of GEIS. At present, GEIS is efficiently run under the direction of the Emerging Disease Program director, but the expansion of NAMRU-2 activities in Indonesia, as well as in other countries, will generate additional responsibilities for the staff. The MoH's new decentralization policy will create a demand for more training and support of national, provincial, and local public health initiatives in Indonesia. GEIS at NAMRU-2 would benefit from a full-time, on-site coordinator possessing, at a minimum, applied epidemiology and public health experience.

The subcommittee was impressed with the high level of staff (DoD, FSN, and contract personnel) commitment to and enthusiasm for GEIS. Staff relationships appeared to be supportive and mutually reinforcing. The committee notes that personnel retention contributes to the formation and enhancement of working relationships and is of particular importance given the emphasis of GEIS on collaborative activities.

NAMRU-2 has worked to promote an extensive collaborative and training role in the Indonesian medical community, and such efforts can be expanded through GEIS. However, training is a time-consuming activity, especially in the absence of a planned, formal training program with a set of organized courses to meet needs for specific skill sets. The subcommittee noted the absence of a training officer to coordinate formal training programs. In addition, no staff are assigned responsibilities for communicating or disseminating surveillance information to other partners.

## TECHNOLOGY AND INFORMATION MANAGEMENT

A tour of the NAMRU-2 facility in Jakarta (including the new BSL-3 space), the warehouse, and the repair shop revealed considerable technical capacity. At the Phnom Penh subsidiary laboratory (under construction), equipment is being procured and installed. A backup generator that will maintain electrical power for all laboratory equipment was in the process of being installed and calibrated. Given current construction and laboratory development efforts, the subcommittee could not assess the available technology in Phnom Penh.

In Jakarta, communications systems provide e-mail, Internet, fax, and telephone access. An on-site data center supplies computer systems support, as well as data entry and analysis services. A separate, but currently overloaded server provides support for the Early Warning Outbreak Response System (EWORS); this server will be upgraded in the near future. In Phnom Penh, communications systems are still under development, although telephone linkages with EWORS sites have been established.

Within the NAMRU-2 laboratory, frozen specimen archives (approximately 300,000 specimens) are maintained and cataloged electronically with an early DOS-based version of the Laboratory Information Tracking System (LITS) software. The U.S. CDC is committed to revising this software in a Windows environment. Although delays have been encountered in the revision, the new software will improve NAMRU-2's ability to store and retrieve data contained in the LITS both in Indonesia and at other field sites.

### Conclusions

In Jakarta, NAMRU-2's technology needs appear to be adequately met for current GEIS operations. Computer and communications technology (access to the World Wide Web, e-mail, library facilities, and an office computer network) appeared to be adequate to support GEIS. In Phnom Penh, plans for equipping the laboratory appear to be sufficient.

## SURVEILLANCE

To understand NAMRU-2's role in infectious disease surveillance in Indonesia, it is important to consider the existing programs and plans of the Ministry of Health and its directorates, which include the Indonesian CDC and Litbangkes. According to the senior adviser to the Minister on Environmental and Disease Control, Indonesian public health priority areas include the World Health Organization (WHO) Expanded Program on Immunization, tuberculosis control (considered to be a very serious problem in Indonesia), malaria, dengue and dengue hemorrhagic fever, human immunodeficiency virus (HIV) infection/AIDS, and pneumonia and diarrhea in children. The adviser also mentioned a current epidemic of human rabies that requires public health attention. Infectious disease surveillance in Indonesia is generally inadequate and is confined to passive reporting. All current NAMRU-2 GEIS surveillance activities depend on sentinel surveillance rather than population-based methods.

The NAMRU-2 GEIS is conceptually organized around the four pillars defined by the GEIS Central Hub. These pillars are

- acute febrile illness surveillance,
- drug-resistant malaria surveillance,
- surveillance for enteric pathogens, and
- influenza surveillance.

All NAMRU-2 GEIS activities are protocol driven, and protocols are defined before any funding is committed.

A great deal of effort was spent to prepare for GEIS implementation and integration of GEIS with national and other partners. Most GEIS projects are in their first year of full funding. Projects funded in fiscal years 2000 to 2004 include continued studies of drug-resistant malaria, influenza surveillance, and drug-resistant enteric bacteria surveillance, as well as projects addressing acute febrile illness and entomological surveillance. Within each pillar, NAMRU-2 has developed several specific projects (NAMRU-2, 2000a).

### *Acute Febrile Illness Surveillance*

The EWORS project addresses the GEIS acute febrile illness surveillance pillar. EWORS was developed by NAMRU-2 and the Indonesian MoH, under the auspices of GEIS, with the objective of sharing surveillance information with the Indonesian government. EWORS is designed to collect standardized data to make area-specific and regional comparisons, to transfer information from network hospitals to a central hub, and to use a syndromic surveillance approach to arrive at a working hypothesis for the observed data (NAMRU-2, undated; NAMRU-2, 2000b). NAMRU-2 staff develop and maintain EWORS software and provide the equipment necessary to support the system.

In Indonesia, the project makes use of eight strategically located sentinel reporting hospitals that provide timely data to identify epidemics. The identification of epidemics, in turn, leads to joint field investigations with the Indonesian CDC and Litbangkes. The eight hospital sites report syndromic data daily to the central EWORS servers, where analysis may identify greater than expected incidences of certain syndromes. In Cambodia, three sentinel sites have been enrolled in EWORS.

EWORS surveillance in Indonesia is limited to patients seeking care from the eight sentinel public health care hospitals. The MoH reported to the subcommittee that previous surveys have indicated that approximately one-third of the Indonesian population seeks care in publicly funded hospitals and that this group probably represents the more disadvantaged segment of the population—the segment most likely to suffer a severe infectious disease burden. The project samples only a portion of the Indonesian population in distinct ecological zones.

Data from EWORS have resulted in a small number of epidemiological and laboratory investigations (e.g., investigation of a dengue outbreak). NAMRU-2 has the flexibility to recognize unusual trends through EWORS and to respond to them. Because the MoH considers EWORS-based surveillance to be extremely important for timely reporting of outbreaks, EWORS computers are being installed directly in both Litbangkes and the Indonesian CDC with linkages to the EWORS server for direct national access to the raw data.

### *Drug-Resistant Malaria Surveillance*

Overall, GEIS goals related to malaria include surveillance, drug resistance monitoring, technology transfer, training of local personnel, and in some instances, provision of supplies and materials to implement specific projects. Clinical and parasitological failures of antimalarial drug therapy will be studied in patients with *Plasmodium falciparum* or *Plasmodium vivax* infections. In an area where a dramatic resurgence of malaria has recently been identified, efforts to train and supply MoH personnel to characterize the epidemics are under way. Included in this GEIS-supported project is a study of primaquine drug resistance.

The long-term goal of this project is the transfer of a sustainable antimalarial drug resistance program to public health authorities in the host country. The combination of MIDRP and GEIS support, and U.S. National Institutes of Health grant funding for surveillance and research to study multiple aspects of malaria parasite microbiology and drug resistance will contribute to national policy formulation, since current standard therapy in Indonesia with chloroquine and pyrimethamine (Fansidar) is often ineffective.

*Surveillance for Enteric Pathogens*

NAMRU-2 has sporadically collected enteric isolates for several years, but now, under the auspices of GEIS, more systematic surveillance efforts are in place. Surveillance sites have been established in seven hospitals (some of which overlap with EWORS sites). These local laboratories isolate and identify a variety of enteric bacteria. Further characterization and antibiotic resistance testing are performed by the NAMRU-2 facility. A variety of enteric pathogens—for example, *Vibrio cholerae*, *Shigella*, *Salmonella*, *Campylobacter*, and *Vibrio parahaemolyticus*—are included in the surveillance activity. In addition, NAMRU-2 staff supported by GEIS provide ongoing training and support to personnel at these sites. In some hospitals, existing laboratories have been strengthened; in others, laboratories for surveillance of enteric pathogens have been established under GEIS.

*Virology and Influenza Surveillance*

The virology laboratory capacity at NAMRU-2 includes tissue culture capabilities along with serological and molecular biological testing technologies. A mix of MIDRP and GEIS funding supports the laboratory infrastructure. Specimens infected with influenza virus are sent to Australia for characterization, and efforts are not closely coordinated with the DoD Laboratory-Based Influenza Surveillance Program, at Brooks Air Force Base, San Antonio, Texas. Influenza surveillance is conducted under the auspices of GEIS through four sentinel specimen collection sites at two different hospitals and primary health care centers for virus isolation and characterization. Surveillance is complicated by the resistance of the Indonesian population to specimen collection that entails the use of nasopharyngeal swabs. In addition, influenza has not been identified as a national priority, although it is a United States and an international priority.

Surveillance activities will be expanded to include a site in Bali, which is a major international travel destination. Basic demographic information will be collected at the time of specimen collection.

## Conclusions

The Indonesian government's laboratory decentralization policy, along with attempts to build both surveillance and laboratory capacity, will bring challenges for NAMRU-2 and GEIS, which may be called upon to provide training for capacity building as well as continuing its current essential support of the MoH.

Improved monitoring of infectious diseases with corresponding epidemic control is a national goal that coincides with the objectives of GEIS. The EWORS project is gathering momentum and is considered extremely important by host-country institutions such as the Indonesian CDC.

Data on health care encounters for febrile syndromes is useful for MoH administrative purposes. Rarely is laboratory follow-up conducted to determine the etiologies of syndromes, however. With additional staffing supported by laboratory diagnostic capacity, the utility of EWORS for the monitoring of emerging infectious diseases would be enhanced.

EWORS will likely not be the only source of information about epidemics. If a more traditional system of surveillance is established in Indonesia, the importance of EWORS may decline (although it is unclear at this time when the infrastructure needed to support such a system would be available). EWORS requires many resources and, as with all syndromic surveillance globally, still needs to be evaluated to better define its usefulness. Regardless, the establishment of a system for the reporting of syndromes and the provision of feedback to the reporting sites will encourage astute clinicians to report unusual events in a timely manner. EWORS is contributing to building the public health infrastructure in Indonesia through strong collaborative ties with key hospitals and the Indonesian CDC and Litbangkes.

GEIS efforts to examine drug-resistant malaria and diseases caused by drug-resistant enteric pathogens are of undeniable importance and are well matched with Indonesian health objectives. NAMRU-2's extensive mosquito insectary capacity is a major asset for the support of studies of malaria. Transfer of entomological expertise to host-country nationals will assist in reestablishing a lost technical capacity in Indonesia and elsewhere for both malaria and dengue.

Improvements in hospital laboratory capacity and the training of locals result from the establishment of enteric pathogen surveillance sites and provide additional benefits for local capacity building. The periodic site visits together with expansion and support of the increased number of sites will result in a vigorous national sentinel surveillance system for diseases caused by enteric pathogens. Dissemination of data to the WHO and other partners for both the prevention and the control of diarrheal diseases will benefit both the host country and the mission of GEIS.

Influenza surveillance at the Indonesian sentinel sites is hampered by lack of acceptance of nasopharyngeal specimen collection techniques. Influenza surveillance may yield better results if it is focused on the U.S. and international communities. GEIS influenza surveillance activities at NAMRU-2 may also benefit from closer collaboration with the Department of Defense Laboratory-Based Influenza Surveillance Program.

There is considerable concordance between national and GEIS objectives, with some notable exceptions. Despite the value of current GEIS surveillance projects, an important surveillance activity is left unaddressed. The subcommittee heard the MoH express concerns about tuberculosis (TB) and multi-drug-resistant TB (MDR-TB)—disease entities that are public health threats on a global basis. Although TB and MDR-TB do not pose an acute threat to deployed military forces, they certainly pose a long-term threat to the health of those forces and U.S. civilians. To the extent that military personnel deployed overseas become infected with *Mycobacterium tuberculosis* or MDR *M. tuberculosis*, the risk to the U.S. civilian population is increased. If it is not brought under control, MDR-TB will continue to pose a threat to U.S. citizens.

The TB program in Indonesia is weak, and many cases of TB go undiagnosed and untreated throughout the country. Laboratories are ill equipped to diagnose and monitor drug resistance. In addition, biosafety concerns are frequently not addressed. The HIV epidemic is just beginning in Indonesia, and cases of TB may arise even more rapidly when the two epidemics intersect. GEIS does not contain a tuberculosis pillar, and GEIS may wish to consider addressing this important global public health issue.

Surveillance data are distributed to national public health authorities and the GEIS Central Hub. Data are also included in the laboratory's annual report and published in peer-reviewed scientific journals. Regular dissemination of NAMRU-2's work to other partners in Indonesia, such as the WHO and the U.S. Agency for International Development (USAID), will enhance partnerships.

The subcommittee questions whether the current annual review and funding process allows sufficient time for surveillance project maturation and planning between reviews. Annual review appears to rush the proposal preparation process and can culminate in the making of decisions about the merits of projects on the basis of incomplete information.

## RESPONSE CAPACITY

The response to epidemics in Indonesia through NAMRU-2 GEIS is carried out at the request of and in collaboration with the Indonesian

CDC and Litbangkes. PACOM and GEIS resources are both important for supporting NAMRU-2 epidemic investigations. National authorities in other countries (e.g., Vietnam, following flooding) have also requested NAMRU-2 collaboration in epidemic investigations. Laboratory support has been provided for investigations of cholera, dengue, anthrax, pertussis, measles, and hepatitis E epidemics in Indonesia and by invitation in Laos and Vietnam. EWORS has also provided training in epidemic investigations for personnel in the host country.

### Conclusions

At NAMRU-2 GEIS possesses resources (e.g., laboratory capacity, staff expertise, and collaborative relationships) that can be and that have been put to use in response to epidemics in Indonesia and in the region. External funding has also been required to support epidemic investigation capacity.

## COLLABORATIONS

GEIS is integrated with current, ongoing activities within Indonesia's public health infrastructure. In-country relationships are largely person based and proximity driven, and strong partnerships have resulted over the years. NAMRU-2 GEIS staff seemed very well known and respected by the national health authorities. The interaction between NAMRU-2 and Litbangkes staff is strong. The MoH, primarily Litbangkes, approves all projects funded by GEIS. GEIS activities are transparent to the Indonesian MoH, and most projects are jointly conducted.

GEIS-funded NAMRU-2 activities serve the Indonesian MoH in important ways, including support of surveillance, assistance with epidemic response, provision of laboratory diagnosis and reference testing services, and training of personnel. NAMRU-2 has offered at-the-bench laboratory training for a variety of national and international personnel. Medical students, residents, and visiting faculty, both national and international, have benefited from time spent at NAMRU-2 in various training modes. NAMRU-2 collaborates closely with AFRIMS, the U.S. CDC, and other international and national institutions both in Indonesia and in Laos, Cambodia, and Vietnam. NAMRU-2 has been designated a WHO Collaborating Center for Emerging Diseases for Southeast Asia (GEIS, 2000e; NAMRU-2, undated).

Collaborative relationships between organizations and agencies with public health interests in Indonesia (including agencies of the Indonesian government, the U.S. government, and international organizations) are quite complex. For example, the subcommittee was advised that the Field

Epidemiology Training Program was located at a university and was not closely linked to the public health mainstream in Indonesia.

Opportunities exist to better leverage the fundamental scientific information generated by GEIS and other NAMRU-2 initiatives with USAID and WHO programming for public health interventions. For example, GEIS has documented the resurgence of malaria in one particular geographical area with considerable ancillary data on drug resistance, parasite type, vectors, and other factors. With financing from USAID and the collaboration of WHO, these data could be used to design a pilot intervention project to control malaria in this region. Results could be scientifically evaluated and the definition of best practices for malaria control in the absence of the use of residual spraying with dichlorodiphenyltrichloroethane (DDT) could make a major contribution to WHO's Roll Back Malaria Program.

### Conclusions

NAMRU-2 staff currently involved with GEIS understand and accommodate the need to establish collaborative and collegial networks within the Indonesian and Cambodian scientific and public health communities, and their efforts to do so are producing many positive results. Special credit needs to be given to the energy and vitality that NAMRU-2 FSN and military staff bring to the program. If GEIS is to be successful, it is important that NAMRU-2 continue its efforts to work through the complex set of relationships that exist within Indonesia to seek and foster productive relationships with other organizations and agencies operating in country. Decentralization will bring the need for closer collaboration with levels of government in Indonesia beyond those with which NAMRU-2 has traditionally shared ties.

The subcommittee noted that there appears to be weak integration of GEIS and the NAMRU-2 capacity with USAID projects, despite NAMRU-2 efforts to engage USAID as a partner. Although USAID is giving high priority to HIV in Indonesia, its local programming could benefit from the public health data generated by GEIS at NAMRU-2. In addition, the WHO's leadership of the multiagency Partners for Health project could also benefit from greater knowledge of GEIS-generated data. Although the WHO office in Jakarta is aware and appreciative of NAMRU-2's contributions, linkages for the sharing of data between these institutions need to be forged and strengthened.

## RECOMMENDATIONS

- GEIS activities at NAMRU-2 are of critical importance to the program as a whole. The committee encourages the DoD to plan for GEIS activities at NAMRU-2 on a long-term basis. NAMRU-2 has already had a substantial impact on Indonesia's public health infrastructure and has contributed to knowledge of emerging infectious diseases. GEIS should be supported in the region even if political exigencies force the withdrawal of NAMRU-2 from Indonesia. NAMRU-2 provides a unique resource for research and for public health missions. Demand for and support of these missions should be balanced so that neither is jeopardized.

**Recommendation: DoD commitment to GEIS at NAMRU-2 should be long term.**

• The coordination of training activities is an important but time-intensive GEIS task. This task needs to be assigned to dedicated personnel responsible for organizing, planning, and administering training activities on a full-time basis. Training local personnel in laboratory technology and epidemic response is an important way in which GEIS can be of benefit in Indonesia. Likewise, training U.S. civilian and military personnel in the NAMRU-2 environment may contribute to meeting GEIS's future recruitment needs as well as to the broader goal of improved global public health surveillance.

**Recommendation: The development of a structured NAMRU-2-hosted training program should be pursued.**

• The reporting of data to Indonesian authorities is being done well. In collaboration with the Indonesian MoH, GEIS should make a more concerted effort to share surveillance information with USAID, the WHO, and other relevant institutions working in Indonesia. Data sharing should be timely and systematic and should be targeted toward achieving effective public health action.

**Recommendation: As GEIS project data are accumulated, they should continue to be used to supplement the national surveillance system and should be better used to help guide public health response through improved sharing of information with international partners, such as the WHO and USAID.**

• NAMRU-2 has established connections with the political and public health infrastructures in Indonesia and understands the subtleties of how to operate effectively in country. NAMRU-2 should continue to strengthen and expand these connections. NAMRU-2 will need to monitor and to be sensitive to the decentralization policy of the MoH. NAMRU-2 may need to modify its GEIS approaches to enhance communication and cooperation at the provincial and district levels. Assistance from the U.S. ambassador should be sought, as needed, to forge alliances with public health partners.

**Recommendation: NAMRU-2 should take continued steps to maintain and enhance the multiple national and international partnerships that are necessary to fulfill the GEIS mission and build national capacity in Indonesia.**

- GEIS development in Cambodia should continue to be supported through close collaboration between NAMRU-2 and AFRIMS.

**Recommendation: NAMRU-2 should continue to support the development of the field laboratory in Cambodia.**

- EWORS is a novel and innovative approach to sentinel surveillance and is one of several surveillance systems that may be useful in Indonesia under a policy of decentralization and reformulation of national surveillance. As a sentinel surveillance system, it needs to be evaluated before decisions are made to greatly expand its use. In addition, greater use of established laboratory capacity to verify the etiology of EWORS-defined syndromes should be initiated to enhance EWORS's utility for the monitoring of emerging infectious diseases.

**Recommendation: EWORS should be evaluated for its capacity to serve as an early-warning system for the detection and investigation of epidemics and for the identification of new and novel pathogens before major investments in expanding the system are made.**

- The current annual approval process does not allow optimal time for project planning or maturation. Furthermore, it is important that the GEIS Central Hub review and approval process for projects provides NAMRU-2 with follow-up guidance regarding project progress in a consistent and timely manner.

**Recommendation: Consideration should be given to revising the current GEIS project application and review process.**

- The subcommittee recognizes that the GEIS pillar disease areas are important ones and that defining these targets helps to provide some standardization of GEIS activities across sites, but the pillar structure should be flexible enough to permit, on a case-by-case basis, local infectious diseases that are of global concern (e.g., tuberculosis) to be addressed as high priorities through GEIS. This serves to take full advantage of the epidemiological setting of the facility, builds national health defenses in the host country, and can be of long-term benefit to the health of many populations, including U.S. military personnel and civilians.

**Recommendation: Consideration should be given to refining the focus of GEIS at NAMRU-2 to better enable diseases outside of the pillar areas to be addressed.**

• Partnerships benefit from knowledge of the local language by senior staff. Partnerships are of increased importance to NAMRU-2 now that its research mission has been expanded to include GEIS activities, which necessitate more interaction with partner agencies. Staff familiarity and comfort with the local language can also improve rates of retention of personnel.

**Recommendation: Senior staff at NAMRU-2 actively involved in GEIS projects should be conversant in the dominant language of the host country or should pursue language training, with the support of GEIS, and should seek to become conversant to the extent possible.**

## PEOPLE MET AND INTERVIEWED

*NAMRU-2 Staff*

CAPT James R. Campbell, commanding officer, NAMRU-2
CDR William K. Alexander, executive officer, NAMRU-2
LT David G. Uwedjojevwe, administrative officer, NAMRU-2
HMC Jesse U. Ladrillono, administrative chief, NAMRU-2
CAPT(Sel) Andrew L. Corwin, director, Emerging Disease Program, NAMRU-2
LT Paul D. Mills, head, LITS, Emerging Disease Program, NAMRU-2
LT John W. Sisson, head, GEIS Emerging Disease Program, NAMRU-2
CDR Kevin R. Porter, director, Viral Disease Program
LT James McArdle, Viral Disease Program
HM2 Gregorio G. Flores, Viral Disease Program
SSG Jonathan W. Sturgis, Viral Disease Program
LCDR B. Anthony Oyofo, director, Bacterial Disease Program, and head, Microbiology Department & Ultrastructure Division
CDR Michael Bangs, head, Entomology Department, Parasitic Disease Program
LCDR Mark D. Lacy, head, Clinical Studies Department, Parasitic Disease Program
HM1 Dennis J. Doolen, Clinical Studies Department, Parasitic Disease Program
LCDR Robert A. Gramzinski, head, Immunology Department, Parasitic Disease Program
LCDR Jason D. Maguire, head, Parasitology Department, Parasitic Disease Program
LT Mazie J. Barcus, head, QA/GCP Department, Parasitic Disease Program

MAJ James W. Boles, head, Laboratory Animal Medicine Department
LCDR Adorado B. Yabut, comptroller
SKCS Aurelio C. Cruz, supply senior chief
HM1 David J. Fontannaz, equipment engineer
Dr. James Olson, assigned to NAMRU-2 from the U.S. Centers for Disease Control and Prevention, National Center for Infectious Diseases

### *NAMRU-2 Associates*

Robert Gelbard, ambassador, United States
Umar F. Achmadi, director general, Indonesian CDC
Sumarjati Arjoso, senior adviser to the Minister on Environmental and Disease Control, Ministry of Health, Republic of Indonesia
Sri Astuti S. Soeparmanto, director, Litbangkes, Department of Health, Ministry of Health, Republic of Indonesia
Jonathan Ross, public health adviser, Office of Population, Health, and Nutrition, U.S. Agency for International Development
Pamela Wolf, senior technical adviser, Office of Population, Health, and Nutrition, U.S. Agency for International Development
Leslie Curtin, director, Office of Population, Health, and Nutrition, U.S. Agency for International Development
Alene Gelbard, senior communications advisor, Office of Population, Health, and Nutrition, U.S. Agency for International Development
Georg Peterson, representative, World Health Organization
Dr. Mam Bunheng, secretary of state for health, Ministry of Health, Kingdom of Cambodia

## ITINERARY

### *Monday, October 2*

Overview presentations regarding GEIS at NAMRU-2. Tour of the NAMRU-2 facility. NAMRU-2 GEIS presentations, including presentations on EWORS, outbreak response activities, enteric surveillance, monitoring, malaria drug resistance, influenza surveillance, and regional surveillance of hemorrhagic diseases.

### *Tuesday, October 3*

Working visits to Litbangkes, Indonesian CDC, and Ministry of Health and other partners and collaborators (i.e., the Thai Field Epidemiology Training Program, USAID, WHO, agency of the host country responsible for epidemiology, collaborating academic partners, etc.), and the U.S. ambassador.

### *Wednesday, October 4*

Continued visits to infectious disease surveillance partners and collaborators. Follow-up meeting(s) with NAMRU-2 staff involved with GEIS projects.

### *Thursday, October 5*

Conclude Jakarta visit. Depart for Bangkok.

### *Friday, October 6*

Travel from Bangkok to Phnom Penh. Meeting with MoH officials. Hospital site visit.

### *Saturday, October 7*

Depart hotel. Return to Bangkok for discussion, drafting of preliminary assessment, and assignment of writing tasks. NAMRU-2 site visit concluded.

# 4

# GEIS at the Armed Forces Research Institute of Medical Sciences, Thailand

The Armed Forces Research Institute of Medical Sciences (AFRIMS) in Bangkok, Thailand, originated in 1959 through an agreement between the governments of the United States and Thailand. The original laboratory was created as the Southeast Asia Treaty Organization's (SEATO's) Cholera Research Laboratory. The laboratory was expanded in 1961 to include research on other tropical diseases and was renamed the SEATO Medical Research Laboratory. SEATO was dissolved in 1977, and the U.S. component of AFRIMS was reorganized as a joint Royal Thai Army–U.S. Army medical research laboratory under the overall command of a Royal Thai Army Officer of flag rank. The U.S. component functions as a special foreign activity of the Walter Reed Army Institute of Research (WRAIR) (GEIS, 2000d). Historically, AFRIMS has been closely linked to and collocated with a Royal Thai Army laboratory. It is physically separated from but collaborates with various other national institutions, including the Thai Ministry of Health (Department of Medical Sciences, National Institute of Health, Department of Communicable Disease Control, and the Office of the Permanent Secretary and its Field Epidemiology Training Program) and the Ministry of Agriculture (Department of Livestock Development).

AFRIMS is probably the most sophisticated diagnostic and research laboratory in all of Southeast Asia. For many years, AFRIMS was devoted exclusively to applied research in support of its medical mission. Research programs with a special emphasis on the development of diagnostic tests and therapeutic products for malaria and other tropical febrile illnesses have been successfully developed. AFRIMS research programs in infectious diseases, including diarrheal disease, malaria vaccine and drug research, viral diseases (specifically, dengue fever and hepatitis), entomology and disease vector research, and retrovirology (including human immunodeficiency virus [HIV] infection/AIDS), existed long before the introduction of the Department of Defense (DoD) Global Emerging Infections Surveillance and Response System (GEIS). In some ways GEIS represents a new departure for AFRIMS, although in other ways GEIS is a natural extension of the field research that has been AFRIMS's mainstay. For example, the GEIS malaria pillar complements ongoing surveillance for antimalarial drug resistance, whereas surveillance for acute febrile illness is a somewhat new area of involvement.

AFRIMS's overall strategy integrates GEIS activities into traditional research streams to leverage AFRIMS resources and expertise already in place, to reduce program overhead costs, and to complement the activities of the Thai government. This integration results in more than 80 percent of GEIS funds being allocated to program implementation rather than overhead costs. In addition, this integration complements and reflects the activities of the Thai government.

AFRIMS's annual budget ranges from $5 million to $7 million and is derived from multiple sources, including the Military Infectious Disease Research Program (MIDRP), HIV prevention and vaccine development programs, the U.S. National Institutes of Health (NIH), various biotechnology and pharmaceutical companies, and the World Health Organization (WHO). GEIS funding for fiscal year 2001, approximately $1,075,000 (GEIS, 2000c), complements these multiple sources of funding. GEIS funding was delayed in the first year of the program, and at the time of the subcommittee's visit, GEIS was in its first full year of funding and many projects were just getting under way.

A subcommittee of the Institute of Medicine (IOM) Committee to Review the Department of Defense (DoD) Global Emerging Infections Surveillance and Response System visited AFRIMS from October 9 to 13, 2000. The IOM subcommittee consisted of committee members Ruth Berkelman, Donald Burke, and Ronald St. John. A list of the people met and interviewed and the itinerary followed can be found at the end of this chapter.

## LABORATORY

AFRIMS has an extensive laboratory facility housed within a 191,000-square-foot laboratory building and animal research unit (GEIS, 2000d). AFRIMS is jointly housed with and shares laboratory space with Royal Thai Army facilities. AFRIMS also occupies a large, modern, extremely well equipped veterinary medicine and animal facility that operates primarily at biosafety level 2. In addition, AFRIMS is linked to approximately 38 field sites in Thailand, Nepal, Vietnam, and Cambodia. AFRIMS supports projects at a Naval Medical Research Unit 2 (NAMRU-2)-maintained subsidiary laboratory in Phnom Penh, Cambodia. This facility provides AFRIMS with an operational base site for additional laboratory and epidemiological studies, including disease surveillance activities.

At AFRIMS, a traditional scientific organizational structure consisting of emerging infectious disease, bacteriology, virology, parasitology, and entomology departments is maintained with extensive capacities in immunology, pharmacology, molecular biology, arthropod culture, and tissue and cell culture. AFRIMS's Bangkok laboratory is equipped to support medical research- and disease surveillance-related activities, activities that use approaches ranging from classical microbiology to modern molecular biology-based approaches. The Association for the Assessment and Accreditation of Laboratory Animal Care–International accredits the laboratory animal facility (GEIS, 2000d). AFRIMS possesses an extensive collection of frozen specimens that are archived in a large number of freezers located throughout the hallways of the laboratory. The specimens are not cataloged centrally through electronic means. Each individual AFRIMS laboratory is responsible for maintaining its own collection.

AFRIMS currently uses its laboratory capacity to support Thailand's infectious disease diagnostic efforts by providing reference testing services, diagnostic support, and support for special epidemic investigations when requested. Thai public health priority areas, along with AFRIMS's training activities, are incorporated into GEIS project areas.

### Conclusions

The laboratory capacity at AFRIMS is sufficient to support current GEIS program activities in Thailand. Nevertheless, AFRIMS laboratories are severely constrained by a lack of adequate laboratory space. All laboratories are severely cramped. Hallways are crowded with freezers housing the extensive collections of specimens maintained by departmental laboratories. There has been little expansion of space over the years, despite the addition of new equipment (e.g., flow cytometers, systems for polymerase chain reaction capacities, etc.) and staff. Technical resources for the laboratory appear adequate, but laboratory space is insufficient.

## STAFFING

At the time of the IOM subcommittee's visit, AFRIMS staff included a total of 306 professional and support personnel (22 U.S. Army staff, 122 foreign service national staff, and 162 contracted personnel). Royal Thai Army staff are not included in this total. In the field, AFRIMS supports 16 nonmilitary staff in Nepal with funding from MIDRP and the NIH. There is no written agreement between the government of Nepal or its national institutions and AFRIMS or the U.S. government acknowledging or providing support for this field station.

FSN staff include senior researchers, laboratory technicians, and contract support personnel, including veterinary and animal care technicians and individuals with expertise in the areas of management and administration.

GEIS is not a department at AFRIMS. Although the GEIS coordinator works within a specific department, GEIS operates as part of the mission of all departments. All department heads have significant involvement in programs other than GEIS, including MIDRP projects. In addition, AFRIMS staff are actively engaged in a multitude of training activities, both formal and informal, for a variety of personnel (laboratory technicians; field survey personnel; and students from the United States and Southeast Asian national and regional institutions, including master's and doctoral candidates, physicians and medical students, and others). Training activities are undertaken without dedicated funding to support the organization and implementation of training activities.[1]

## Conclusions

At AFRIMS, GEIS benefits from a dedicated, skilled scientific team, but there is little expertise in epidemiology and public health. The GEIS coordinator needs to possess experience and extensive applied epidemiology and public health expertise for GEIS to reach its objectives. Regional expansion of AFRIMS's activities in Thailand, as well as in other countries in Southeast Asia, will generate additional responsibilities for the GEIS coordinator. Training needs at the national and regional levels are likely to continue in the future.

The subcommittee was impressed with staff members' (DoD, FSN, and contract personnel) commitment to and enthusiasm for GEIS projects. Staff relationships appeared to be supportive and mutually reinforcing. The committee notes that retention of personnel contributes to the formation and enhancement of working relationships and is of particular importance given the emphasis of GEIS on collaborative activities.

[1]Training for national, international, and U.S. personnel is compatible with the Presidential Directive, that is, "Expand formal training and outreach to health care providers" (NSTC, Executive Office of the President, 1996).

## TECHNOLOGY AND INFORMATION MANAGEMENT

A tour of the AFRIMS facility in Bangkok, including the renovated veterinary medicine and animal facility, revealed considerable technical capacity. Communications systems provide e-mail, Internet, fax, and telephone access. An on-site data center supplies computer systems support, as well as data entry and analysis services.

### Conclusions

In Bangkok, AFRIMS's technology needs appear to be adequately met for current GEIS operations. Computer and communications technology (access to the World Wide Web, e-mail, library facilities, and an office computer network) appeared adequate to support GEIS. In Phnom Penh, plans for equipping the laboratory appear to be sufficient.

The introduction of computer-based uniform cataloging software would improve AFRIMS's ability to store and retrieve the data and specimens contained in its extensive collection.

## SURVEILLANCE

At AFRIMS GEIS includes four standard pillars defined by the GEIS Central Hub (AFRIMS, 2000). These pillars are

- drug-resistant malaria surveillance,
- surveillance for enteric pathogens and antibiotic resistance,
- acute febrile illness surveillance, and
- influenza surveillance.

AFRIMS has developed several specific projects within each pillar. In addition, AFRIMS has developed veterinary medicine projects (zoonotic disease surveillance) with GEIS funding. In the conduct of these studies (e.g., studies of leptospirosis), GEIS-supported staff work closely with the Thai Ministry of Agriculture. AFRIMS has also developed extensive expertise for the study of scrub typhus, a commonly encountered cause of febrile illness in Thailand. AFRIMS has under way studies of both the vector and the rickettsial agent of scrub typhus.

Thailand's network of regional and local hospitals provides an extensive infrastructure for infectious disease reporting. AFRIMS does not play a major role in the Thai national surveillance system and thus is not involved in the day-to-day management of infectious disease programs including epidemic investigations. Through joint collaborations, common research studies, and a long history of mutual assistance, Thai public health authorities have come to value AFRIMS's expertise and unique capabilities in specific infectious diseases, especially malaria. AFRIMS's contributions are uniquely suited to meet the specific needs of individual countries in the Southeast Asian region.

AFRIMS has made a conscious decision to concentrate GEIS field activities in border areas (especially in the west, along the Thai-Myanmar [Burma] border) because the Thai Ministry of Public Health has extensive surveillance coverage and health care service delivery capacities in the more central geographical areas of the country and because large numbers of displaced individuals, including refugees, are located in these areas. AFRIMS's infectious disease surveillance activities are generated by specific study protocols and are generally limited to patients seeking care at public and nongovernmental (missionary) health care facilities. The subcommittee did not ascertain the proportion of the Thai population that is estimated to seek care in publicly funded or missionary hospitals. Presumably, this segment of the population represents the more disadvantaged segment that is most likely to suffer a severe burden of infectious disease. GEIS projects sample only a portion of the Thai population in distinct ecological zones. All current GEIS surveillance activities depend on sentinel surveillance rather than population-based methods. Sentinel surveillance is, however, a reasonable approach for a supplemental surveillance activity such as GEIS.

*Drug-Resistant Malaria Surveillance*

AFRIMS's malaria research program is long-standing and internationally recognized. Funds from multiple sources support a variety of projects. The largest funding source is MIDRP. AFRIMS's malaria research program is well situated in Thailand, where all four vectors and malaria species are present and significant drug resistance occurs. AFRIMS carries out extensive surveillance and testing for drug-resistant strains. As a result, AFRIMS has traditionally participated in the development and field testing of new therapeutic agents (e.g., tafenoquine) and combination therapies (e.g., mefloquine-artesunate). In addition, basic research on malaria vaccine candidates as an alternative to therapeutic and prophylactic drugs continues. Malaria research at AFRIMS is backed up with an extensive insectary and entomological expertise. Studies are conducted in multiple field sites along the northwest border with Myanmar and the eastern border with Cambodia, as well as in the Hospital for Tropical Diseases at Mahidol University in Bangkok. In addition, field sites exist in Vietnam, Nepal, and Bangladesh.

The malaria surveillance and research effort is a single integrated program, and GEIS funding is used to support its ongoing surveillance for resistant strains. In addition, GEIS efforts in acute febrile illness surveillance are piggybacked on the infrastructure created at malaria field sites. This integration was clearly demonstrated for the subcommittee during the field visit to the Sangkhlaburi study site in rural Thailand, along the Myanmar border.

*Surveillance for Enteric Pathogens and Antibiotic Resistance*

AFRIMS has sporadically collected enteric isolates for several years, but now, under the auspices of GEIS, more systematic surveillance efforts are being developed by a recently appointed director for this activity. Enhancement of surveillance activities for enteric pathogens, improvement of the local laboratory infrastructure, and tracking of antibiotic resistance patterns are all program goals. Laboratory capacity includes molecular genetics capabilities. Case-control studies in Thailand (at three sites, including locations involved in the military exercise Operation Cobra Gold), Vietnam, and Nepal have identified *Salmonella, Shigella* enterotoxigenic *Escherichia coli*, and *Campylobacter* as common pathogens. Isolate characterization and antibiotic resistance testing are performed by the AFRIMS facility. Specimens from cholera epidemics have also been collected. Additional sentinel surveillance sites in Thailand, Nepal, and Vietnam are planned. The criteria used to select these sentinel sites include access to travelers, ease of implementation, and use of existing field sites. Of six proposed enteric pathogen surveillance projects, three are currently funded.

*Acute Febrile Illness Surveillance*

Surveillance for acute febrile illness is based in sentinel surveillance sites that were established previously for other projects, such as long-standing antimalarial drug resistance surveillance sites. New sites (e.g., Chiang Rai Hospital) are being developed with GEIS funding.

GEIS-coordinated acute febrile illness surveillance recently began at the Kamphaeng Phet Provincial Hospital, which has been a virology-dengue sentinel site since the 1980s. The records of hospitalized patients are reviewed daily for dengue-like illness, encephalitis, hemorrhagic fever or sepsis, febrile respiratory infection, hepatitis or jaundice, malaria, and unexplained sudden death. Nevertheless, surveillance is passive, with no proactive component for a quick response to trends in specific syndromes. Reports of syndromes appear to be analyzed months after they are reported, thus limiting the opportunity for timely epidemiological investigation and providing little opportunity for specimen collection and accurate diagnosis.

The subcommittee visited the malaria-acute febrile illness sentinel surveillance site in Sangkhlaburi, a small town in the tropical rain forest very close to the Myanmar border in western Thailand. The site is located in an established missionary hospital serving a predominantly rural and displaced population living along the border. Surveillance is set up to evaluate the incidence of emerging diseases in febrile patients in both the inpatient and outpatient settings. This sentinel site has documented a significant incidence of leptospirosis among febrile patients. These patients had previously been misdiagnosed with malaria. Malaria, leptospirosis,[2] and undifferentiated pneumonia are common diagnoses confirmed by the AFRIMS laboratory on site. A significant proportion of all fever cases are undiagnosed, on the basis of AFRIMS and missionary hospital data.

### *Virology and Influenza Surveillance*

The virology laboratory capacity at AFRIMS is extensive for specific viral entities, including flavivirus (the agent of dengue) and hepatitis viruses. AFRIMS's virological capacity and interests go well beyond the goals of GEIS. A mixture of MIDRP and GEIS funding supports the virology laboratory infrastructure.

Influenza surveillance is conducted as part of the DoD Laboratory-Based Influenza Surveillance Program, Brooks Air Force Base, San Antonio, Texas. GEIS-supported sentinel sites for specimen collection exist in Nepal and Thailand. Emphasis is on the collection of specimens from travelers and trekkers who acquire influenza viruses through their travels. Specimens are sent to Brooks Air Force Base for processing. Only 39 specimens from Thailand and Nepal had been collected at the time of the subcommittee's visit. A Thai influenza laboratory, linked to the WHO Influenza Collaborating Reference Laboratory in Australia, conducts separate influenza surveillance activities. The Thai laboratory has collected more than 100 specimens for processing through the WHO system.

## Conclusions

There is considerable concordance between Thai national and GEIS objectives, with some notable exceptions. Thai public health authorities often mentioned tuberculosis (TB) and multi-drug-resistant TB (MDR-TB) as serious national concerns. Although MDR-TB does not pose an acute threat to deployed military forces, it certainly poses a long-term threat to the health of those forces and U.S. civilians. To the extent that military personnel deployed overseas become infected with MDR *Mycobacterium*

[2]According to AFRIMS, 27 percent of the patients with fever and rash were diagnosed with leptospirosis.

*tuberculosis*, the risk to the U.S. civilian population is increased. If it is not brought under control, MDR-TB will continue to pose a threat to U.S. citizens. The current GEIS does not contain a tuberculosis pillar, and GEIS may wish to address this important global public health issue.

GEIS efforts to examine drug-resistant malaria and drug-resistant enteric disease pathogens are of undeniable importance and are well matched with Thai health objectives. The combination of MIDRP, GEIS, NIH, WHO, and pharmaceutical company funding for malaria surveillance and research supports projects that will contribute to national health policy formulation, as well as to the global WHO Roll Back Malaria Program, and military health objectives.

Surveillance of antimicrobial resistance in enteric pathogens is just beginning, and linkages to the Ministry of Health to share the resulting data are needed. Timely sharing of surveillance results is important for the development of informed national policies for human, animal, and agricultural antibiotic use. AFRIMS staff, supported by GEIS, provide considerable training in the course of establishing enteric pathogen sentinel sites in the Southeast Asian region. Improvements in hospital laboratory capacity also result from the establishment of enteric pathogen surveillance sites and contribute to the building of local public health capacity.

Syndromic surveillance is a valuable tool for rapid decision making; however, it requires timely investigation and laboratory diagnosis to confirm the etiologies of the syndromes. Epidemiological investigation of unusual trends in acute febrile syndromes, along with active feedback of surveillance results to the reporting institutions, is necessary to establish a robust system for detection of unusual events. Timely analysis of trends in syndromic surveillance, coupled with laboratory diagnosis and strong interactions with the reporting institutions, may create an environment in which rapid notification of an unusual event by an astute clinician will occur.

The initial work at Sangkhlaburi on acute febrile illness with AFRIMS laboratory support is exemplary. Data from GEIS acute febrile illness surveillance efforts have resulted in epidemiological and laboratory investigations into new areas (e.g., leptospirosis and scrub typhus in both Thailand and Cambodia). The results of this program can aid in development and treatment efforts in Thailand and the region.

However, acute febrile illness surveillance efforts would benefit from a reevaluation of project goals. If the purpose is to find a previously unknown pathogen, protocols to study specific syndromes need to be developed. For example, at the Sangkhlaburi and Kamphaeng Phet Hospitals, a significant proportion of the patients present with a pulmonary infection syndrome, but no specific protocol has been developed to pursue a laboratory diagnosis in this subgroup. Similarly, other acute febrile syndromes could be explored one by one. On the other hand, if the overall purpose of the surveillance is to evaluate rapid methods for the detection of multiple disease agents (e.g., Dip-S-Ticks, currently in use) or to identify persons infected or colonized with known pathogens for further study of risk factors associated with their illness, then other types of studies are required.

Influenza surveillance as currently structured in Bangkok may be redundant in the presence of a WHO collaborating laboratory in Thailand. Focusing specimen collection efforts on other populations not sampled by the WHO collaborating laboratory, for example populations of travelers, trekkers in Nepal, and U.S. Embassy personnel, may more effectively supplement the surveillance conducted by the national center.

The subcommittee also questions whether the current annual review and funding process allows sufficient time for surveillance project maturation and planning between reviews. Annual review appears to rush the proposal preparation process and can culminate in the making of decisions about the merits of projects on the basis of incomplete information.

## RESPONSE CAPACITY

AFRIMS participation in response efforts in Thailand is usually requested only when AFRIMS specialized expertise or capabilities are needed. AFRIMS GEIS response to epidemics in Thailand is usually carried out in collaboration with the Thai Department of Communicable Disease Control (Thai CDC) and the Thai Field Epidemiology Training Program (FETP). National authorities in other countries have also requested AFRIMS collaboration in investigations of epidemics. AFRIMS has collaborated in identifying the causative pathogens in several epidemics of acute febrile illness.

As GEIS project data accumulate, ongoing epidemiological analyses of these data may be used to identify unusual events and possible epidemics.

### Conclusions

At AFRIMS GEIS possesses unique resources (e.g., laboratory capacity, staff expertise, and collaborative relationships) that can be and that have been put to use in response to epidemics in Thailand and in the region.

## COLLABORATIONS

To understand AFRIMS's role in infectious disease surveillance in Thailand, it is important to consider the existing programs and plans of the Ministry of Health and its relevant components, that is, the Department of Medical Sciences (DMS), which includes the National Institute of Health; the Thai CDC; and the Office of the Permanent Secretary, which houses the Field Epidemiology Training Program. In addition, the Ministry of Agriculture's Department of Livestock Development is an important collaborating institution.

Steps have been taken to integrate GEIS with current, ongoing activities within Thailand's public health infrastructure. In-country relationships are person based as well as position based, and strong partnerships have resulted over the years. GEIS-funded AFRIMS activities serve the Thai Ministry of Health in important ways, including support of surveillance, assistance with epidemic response, provision of laboratory diagnosis and reference testing services, and training of personnel. AFRIMS has offered at-the-bench laboratory training for a variety of national and international personnel. Medical and public health students, residents, and visiting faculty—national and international—have benefited from time spent at AFRIMS in various training modes. AFRIMS collaborates closely with NAMRU-2, the U.S. Centers for Disease Control and Prevention (U.S. CDC), and other international and national institutions both in Thailand as well as in Nepal, Cambodia, and Vietnam.

According to the director general of the DMS, Paijit Warachit, Thai Ministry of Health priority areas are, first and foremost, HIV infection, malaria, and tuberculosis. Other priority areas include dengue, encephalitis, leptospirosis, diarrheal diseases, and emerging infectious diseases, especially those that cross land borders. Thailand is completing the fifth year of its Eighth National Health Plan and will shortly begin a new 5-year plan (the ninth). The new plan contemplates the merging of the Thai CDC, the Office of Epidemiology (Office of Permanent Secretary), and the DMS into a single program area. AFRIMS is seen as a potential collaborator with the Thai Ministry of Health emerging infectious disease program in light of its expertise and its linkages with other international laboratory networks. Previous collaboration has been ad hoc and project oriented, although opportunities for more structured collaboration may arise. Laboratory support for surveillance (e.g., to help process specimens from the Mekong Malaria project), assistance with building a national laboratory capacity, information exchange, and facilitation of linkages to international laboratory expertise were areas identified for AFRIMS collaboration with the DMS and the Thai CDC. There appeared to be good relations with the U.S. CDC field station located near the Thai CDC; however, there was relatively little collaboration with AFRIMS, although the committee notes that the U.S. CDC is planning to expand its involvement in Thailand as part of a new U.S. CDC initiative (Dowell, 2001).

Linkages between AFRIMS GEIS acute febrile illness surveillance activities and national epidemic investigation capacity were not clear. For instance, the relationship between AFRIMS and the established Thai FETP and the Mekong Malaria project, involving epidemiological collaborations between among the six nations joined by the Mekong River, was unclear. In a conversation between one of the IOM subcommittee members (R. St. John) and Somsak Wattanasri, current director of the Ministry of Health's International Health Office and former director of the Thai FETP in the Office of the Permanent Secretary, it was noted that ties with AFRIMS were much stronger in the past. Since FETP moved to the main Ministry of Health complex in Nonthaburi, some distance from the center of the city, the level of FETP-AFRIMS collaboration appears to have declined significantly.

Strong traditional linkages exist with the research departments at WRAIR and various U.S. academic institutions. There are ongoing collaborations with multiple laboratories in both the academic and private sectors in such areas as antimalarial drug research. Ongoing relationships with academic institutions continue to provide AFRIMS with substantial expertise. AFRIMS has a long-standing collaboration with the Harvard School of Public Health for studies of *Ehrlichia* spp. Other institutions have collaborated in many research studies of dengue.

Although AFRIMS has the flexibility required to recognize many but not all new pathogens identified through sentinel surveillance networks, with the broad variety of pathogenic agents encountered in Southeast Asia, the staff expressed an ongoing need to identify additional institutions with unique in-depth expertise in the detection of emerging pathogens. From time to time, AFRIMS may require in-depth expertise from outside sources. For example, the laboratory identification of strains of *Leptospira* (the agent of leptospirosis) is sometimes difficult, and additional expertise available in other U.S. institutions may be required. Additional linkages with other institutions for in-depth expert support would facilitate rapid collaboration for the identification of unusual pathogens.

## Conclusions

AFRIMS staff currently involved with GEIS understand and accommodate the need to establish collaborative and collegial networks with the Thai, Nepalese, Vietnamese, and Cambodian scientific and public health communities, and their efforts to do so are producing many positive results.

The collaborative relationships between and among organizations and agencies with public health interests in Thailand (including agencies of the Thai government, the U.S. government, and international organizations) are quite complex. Additional opportunities exist to share the fundamental scientific information generated by GEIS and other AFRIMS initiatives with institutions in the host country (e.g., in the area of enteric pathogens) and to strengthen relationships between AFRIMS and the Thai CDC and FETP.

If GEIS is to be successful, AFRIMS must continue to work through the complex set of relationships that exist within Thailand and continue to work with other in-country international organizations and agencies on a continual and productive basis. Satellite laboratories and sentinel surveillance sites in Southeast Asia are most likely to operate efficiently and effectively if GEIS efforts are coordinated among GEIS consortium members in the region (including AFRIMS, NAMRU-2, and the 18th Medical Command in Korea).

AFRIMS has worked to promote an extensive collaborative and training role in the Thai medical community, and such efforts can be expanded through GEIS. However, training for GEIS-related projects can be time-consuming, especially in the absence of a planned, formal training program with a set of organized courses to meet needs for specific skill sets. The subcommittee noted the absence of a training officer to coordinate formal training programs.

## RECOMMENDATIONS

- GEIS activities at AFRIMS are of critical importance to GEIS as a whole. The committee encourages the DoD to plan for GEIS activities at AFRIMS on a long-term basis. AFRIMS provides a unique resource for research and for public health missions. Demand for and support of these missions should be balanced so that neither is jeopardized.

**Recommendation: DoD commitment to GEIS at AFRIMS should be long term.**

- Data obtained from GEIS projects should be evaluated and, where useful, reported to Thai authorities and other relevant institutions working in Thailand and Southeast Asian countries, as well as regional WHO offices. Reporting should be timely and systematic and should be targeted toward achieving effective public health action.

**Recommendation: As GEIS project data are accumulated, they should be better used to supplement national and regional surveillance systems and to help guide public health responses through improved reporting to authorities in the host country.**

- AFRIMS has established connections with the political and public health infrastructures in Thailand and understands the subtleties of how to operate effectively in country. AFRIMS should continue to strengthen and expand these connections and take steps to overcome the geographical separation of GEIS from the Thai Ministry of Health. In particular, AFRIMS should consider reestablishing stronger ties with FETP, which can serve as a link to multinational surveillance and epidemic investigation efforts, such as the Mekong Malaria project. Assistance from the regional unified combatant command and the U.S. ambassador should be sought, as needed.

**Recommendation: AFRIMS should continue to take steps to maintain and enhance the multiple national and international partnerships that are necessary to fulfill the GEIS mission.**

• The subcommittee recognizes that the GEIS pillar disease areas are important ones and that defining these targets helps to provide some standardization of GEIS activities across sites, but the pillar structure should be flexible enough to permit, on a case-by-case basis, local infectious diseases that are of global concern (e.g., tuberculosis) to be addressed as high priorities through GEIS. This serves to take full advantage of the epidemiological setting of the facility, builds national health defenses in the host country, and can be of long-term benefit to the health of many populations, including U.S. military personnel and civilians.

**Recommendation: Consideration should be given to refining the focus of GEIS at AFRIMS to better enable diseases outside of the pillar areas to be addressed.**

• To avoid duplication of efforts and to fully benefit from existing capabilities, all GEIS activities in Southeast Asia (e.g., those GEIS activities maintained by AFRIMS, NAMRU-2, and the 18th Medical Command) should be closely coordinated.

**Recommendation: AFRIMS GEIS efforts should be coordinated with the efforts of other DoD facilities (i.e., laboratories, the GEIS Central Hub, and other GEIS partners) that host GEIS projects in the region.**

**Recommendation: To fully realize GEIS objectives, AFRIMS should have a full-time, on-site GEIS program manager who possesses expertise in applied epidemiology and public health.**

• Current approaches to influenza surveillance in Thailand may require revision to avoid duplication of effort with laboratories that currently participate in the WHO influenza surveillance network. Influenza surveillance would be more fruitful if it was coordinated with laboratories that currently participate in the WHO influenza surveillance system to avoid duplicate sampling of the same populations. AFRIMS surveillance could concentrate on different populations not sampled by the WHO site, such as travelers seeking care in U.S. Embassy facilities in Thailand, Nepal, and other countries.

**Recommendation: Influenza surveillance efforts should be coordinated with the Thai WHO collaborating laboratory.**

• The coordination of training activities is an important but time-intensive task of GEIS. This task should be assigned to dedicated personnel whose full-time responsibility is the organizing, planning, and administration of training activities. Training of local personnel in laboratory technology is an important way in which GEIS can be of benefit in Thailand. Likewise, because AFRIMS capabilities are unique, training of U.S. civilian and military personnel in the AFRIMS environment may contribute to meeting GEIS's future recruitment needs, as well as training needs within the DoD and public health community more generally.

**Recommendation: The development of a structured AFRIMS-hosted training program should be considered.**

• Partnerships benefit from knowledge of the local language by senior staff. Partnerships are of increased importance to AFRIMS now that its research mission has been expanded to include GEIS activities, which necessitate more interaction with partner agencies. Staff familiarity and comfort with the local language can also improve rates of retention of personnel.

**Recommendation: Senior staff at AFRIMS actively involved in GEIS projects should be conversant in the dominant language of the host country or should pursue, with the support of GEIS, language training, and should seek to become conversant to the extent possible.**

• The current annual approval process does not allow optimal time for AFRIMS project planning or maturation. Furthermore, it is important that the GEIS Central Hub review and approval process for GEIS projects provides AFRIMS with follow-up guidance regarding project progress in a consistent and timely manner (see also Chapter 7).

**Recommendation: Consideration should be given to revising the current GEIS project application and review process.**

## PEOPLE MET AND INTERVIEWED

### *AFRIMS Staff*

COL G. Dennis Shanks
MAJ Gaye Ruble
LTC Art Brown
MAJ (P) Russ Coleman

LTC Carl Mason
LTC Timothy Endy
LTC David Ruble
MAJ R. Scott Miller
Chansuda Wonsrichanalai
MG Gobchoke (Royal Thai Army)

*AFRIMS Associates*

Ambassador Richard Hecklinger, United States
Dr. Rapeegong Vongdee, director general, Ministry of Agriculture
Dr. Paijit Warachit, deputy director general, Department of Medical Sciences, Ministry of Public Health
Dr. Supamit, director, Division of General Communicable Disease
Dr. Kamnuan, director, FETP
Dr. Sonchai, dean, Faculty of Tropical Medicine, Mahidol University
Dr. Pathom Sawanpanyalert, director, Department of Medical Sciences, National Institute of Health, Ministry of Public Health
Dr. Sornchai Looareesuwan, dean, Faculty of Tropical Medicine, Mahidol University
Dr. Punnee Pitisuttithum, Vaccine Trial Center, Faculty of Tropical Medicine, Mahidol University
Dr. Srivicha Krudsood, Department of Tropical Hygiene, Faculty of Tropical Medicine, Mahidol University
Dr. Somsak Wattansari, director, International Health Office, Ministry of Public Health

## ITINERARY

*Monday, October 9*

0800 Depart hotel
0800 Meet with Dr. Rapeegong, Ministry of Agriculture
1030 Group meeting at the Ministry of Public Health
Dr. Paijit, deputy director general, Department of Medical Sciences
Dr. Supamit, Director, Division of General Communicable Disease
Dr. Kamnuan, Director, FETP
1230 Lunch
1400 Meet with Dr. Sonchai, dean, Faculty of Tropical Medicine, Mahidol University
1630 Return to hotel

### *Tuesday, October 10*

| | |
|---|---|
| 0800 | Depart hotel |
| 0830 | Arrive at AFRIMS; meet with AFRIMS commander, MG Gobchoke, RTA |
| 0900 | IOM in brief |
| 0915 | USAMC-AFRIMS Commander, COL Dennis Shanks–overview of AFRIMS/mission |
| 0945 | AFRIMS-GEIS overview, MAJ Gaye Ruble |
| 1015 | Break |
| 1030 | Department briefs (30–45 minutes each)<br>Retrovirology—LTC Art Brown<br>Entomology—MAJ (P) Russ Coleman<br>Enterics—LTC Carl Mason<br>Virology—LTC Timothy Endy |
| 1215 | Lunch (at AFRIMS, room 302)—XO, officers, Thai scientists |
| 1330 | Depart for U.S. Embassy (IOM team, COL Shanks, MAJ Ruble) |
| 1430 | Meet with Ambassador Hecklinger |
| 1515 | Depart U.S. Embassy |
| 1600 | Return to hotel |

### *Wednesday, October 11*

| | |
|---|---|
| 0800 | Depart hotel |
| 0830 | Arrive AFRIMS<br>Finish departmental briefs and tour facility<br>Entomology<br>Immunology<br>Enterics<br>Virology<br>Retrovirology (time permitting) |
| 1130 | Lunch and depart for Sangkhlaburi (LTC Ruble, MAJ (P) Miller, MAJ Ruble, and IOM team) |
| 1830 | Arrive Sangkhlaburi |

### *Thursday, October 12*

| | |
|---|---|
| 0800 | Immunology brief, MAJ (P) Scott Miller<br>Veterinary medicine brief, LTC David Ruble |
| 0930 | Tour hospital, villages<br>Meet with local collaborators |
| 1200 | Lunch |

Depart Sangkhlaburi
1900 Arrive Bangkok

***Friday, October 13***

0800 Depart hotel
0830 Arrive AFRIMS
Final questions for AFRIMS staff
0900 Private IOM discussions; IOM out-brief, official good-byes

# 5

# GEIS at Naval Medical Research Unit 3, Egypt

Naval Medical Research Unit 3 (NAMRU-3), is the largest U.S. military medical research facility operating overseas and one of the largest medical research laboratories in the North Africa-Middle East region. The laboratory traces its origins back to 1942, when American scientists and technicians began working with Egyptian physicians at the Abassia Fever Hospital, Cairo, Egypt, under the auspices of the U.S. Typhus Commission, established by President Franklin D. Roosevelt.

After World War II, the Egyptian government invited the U.S. Navy to continue collaborative studies of endemic tropical and subtropical diseases with Egyptian scientists. NAMRU-3 was formally established in 1946, and the laboratory has been in continuous operation ever since, despite periods of political tension and a 7-year lapse in U.S.–Egyptian relations (from 1967 to 1973). For a short period, NAMRU-3 had a satellite facility in Ethiopia (which operated for a time as NAMRU-5), but the facility was closed because of political difficulties. NAMRU-3 is hosted by the Egyptian Ministry of Health and Population (MOHP) and has worked closely with the MOHP and the Abbasia Fever Hospital for over 50 years.

Though NAMRU-3 has historically been dedicated to a research mission, infectious disease surveillance and response activities were conducted at NAMRU-3 before the introduction of GEIS. GEIS has supported surveillance projects at NAMRU-3 since 1998 (NAMRU-3, 2000a). GEIS support for NAMRU-3 surveillance projects totaled $1,000,000 in fiscal year 2000 (GEIS, 2000b) and is expected to total $1,075,000 in fiscal year 2001 (GEIS, 2000c).

A subcommittee of the Institute of Medicine (IOM) Committee to

Review the Department of Defense Global Emerging Infections Surveillance and Response System visited NAMRU-3 from October 8 to 14, 2000. The subcommittee consisted of committee members Kathleen Gensheimer, James Hospedales, and Guénaël Rodier. A list of the people who the subcommittee met with and the itinerary that was followed can be found at the end of this chapter.

## LABORATORY

NAMRU-3 has extensive laboratory capacities, particularly in virology but also in bacteriology and parasitology. NAMRU-3 also maintains extensive insectary and animal research facilities. The animal research facility is accredited by the Association for Assessment and Accreditation of Laboratory Animal Care-International (GEIS, 2000f).

NAMRU-3 headquarters are housed within 68,000 square feet of laboratory space, 25,000 square feet of office space, 9,200 square feet of warehouse and supply storage space, and 2,750 square feet of biosafety level 3 biocontaminant space in Cairo, Egypt (GEIS, 2000f). Field sites are maintained in Abu Homos (for the study of enteric pathogens) and Qus and Armut (for the study of febrile illnesses), Egypt.

### Conclusions

The value of NAMRU-3 laboratory capacities is widely acknowledged by all public health partners, such as the MOHP. NAMRU-3 facilities play an essential role in supporting operational research in infectious diseases and infectious disease surveillance in Egypt and in the region. Such capabilities constitute the basis for the close partnership and working relations between NAMRU-3 and the Egyptian MOHP, the World Health Organization (WHO) Regional Office for the Eastern Mediterranean (EMRO), and the U.S. Agency for International Development (USAID). The laboratory capacity is clearly sufficient to support the mission of the Global Emerging Infections Surveillance and Response System (GEIS).

## STAFFING

NAMRU-3 is organized into administrative and research departments. Virology Research, Disease Surveillance, Enteric Disease Research, and Vector Biology Research Programs are maintained within NAMRU-3's Research Sciences Department (RSD). GEIS is coordinated by the director of the RSD. GEIS plays a major role in supporting the newly created NAMRU-3 Disease Surveillance Program (supported with a combination of GEIS and USAID funds) and significantly contributes to the Virology

Research Program and the Enteric Diseases Research Program. GEIS provides little or no support for the Vector Biology Research Program.

At the time of the IOM subcommittee's visit, NAMRU-3 staff included 40 military assignees; among them were 20 professional, uniformed services personnel (17 U.S. Navy, 2 U.S. Army, and 1 U.S. Public Health Service, Centers for Disease Control and Prevention [CDC] personnel). In addition, NAMRU-3 employs a staff of approximately 141 foreign service nationals (FSNs). The deputy director of RSD is an FSN with long-term service with NAMRU-3 and plays a key role in the continuity and institutional memory of NAMRU-3 and in maintaining relationships with collaborators, particularly the Egyptian MOHP. No full-time employee works exclusively on GEIS projects. All department heads have significant involvement in programs other than GEIS.

At the time of the subcommittee visit, layoffs of FSN employees were anticipated before the end of 2000. Layoffs were to occur as the result of financial limitations and a decision to outsource more services. These anticipated layoffs resulted in some concern among staff that NAMRU-3 may not be able maintain operations at current levels.

## Conclusions

NAMRU-3 hosts a dedicated, skilled scientific team that can fulfill the objectives of GEIS. Staff relationships appeared to be supportive and mutually reinforcing. At present, GEIS is efficiently administered by the director of the RSD, but there is no overall oversight of GEIS by individuals or organizational units with expertise in epidemiology. GEIS at NAMRU-3 would benefit from a full-time, on-site coordinator possessing, at a minimum, applied epidemiology and public health experience.

Although a high level of commitment to GEIS was observed and GEIS has been given strong support from the CDC assignee who directs the Disease Surveillance Program, the organizational structure of the RSD does not formally put the Disease Surveillance Program in a position to coordinate surveillance activities and data or to foster collaboration between projects and among programs. A shortage of military public health personnel with a sufficient background in applied epidemiology and disease surveillance also appeared to be of concern. In particular, there did not appear to be a full understanding of the public health implications of the GEIS mission, including the need to strengthen the capacities of countries in the region.

A strength of GEIS at NAMRU-3 is the presence of FSN staff who play a key role not only in the management and technical support of GEIS but also in the integration of the program with other in-country infectious disease surveillance activities and in the improvement of ties with NAMRU-3's partners in public health activities. Because of their potential for long-term service, the involvement of FSNs with the efforts of NAMRU-3 is integral to the full implementation and continuity of the GEIS mission. Continuity in the senior management of NAMRU-3 is also important to the fulfillment of the GEIS mission. Although retention of military personnel is probably not a concern unique to NAMRU-3, the potential for military staff turnover to disrupt the GEIS mission poses a very real concern.

## TECHNOLOGY AND INFORMATION MANAGEMENT

A tour of the NAMRU-3 facility in Cairo revealed considerable technical capacity, including access to the Internet (to be further improved), e-mail, library facilities, and a local area network. A visit to the Abu Homos study site on the Nile delta (Enteric Diseases Research Program) showed good information technology (IT) facilities, whereas sites at Armut in Upper Egypt (cohort and sentinel studies carried out by the Disease Surveillance Program) showed more limited IT facilities.

NAMRU-3 maintains two different laboratory information systems. A "homegrown," ACCESS (database)-based specimen registration system (the LISA system) has been developed to catalog all but virology specimens. The LISA system is a stand-alone system and does not extend to the computerization of testing in the various laboratories, nor does it support the reporting of results or the analysis of aggregate data patterns and trends. The second system, a virology system, was not reviewed but is understood to be a Paradox (database)-based, separate system for accessioning of virology specimens. As for the LISA system, this system does not extend to the computerization of testing in the various laboratories or report results.

An overall plan to integrate NAMRU-3 information facilities, including IT-related hardware and software, communications activities, information feedback activities, and dissemination efforts, does not exist. NAMRU-3 surveillance-related information is disseminated through quarterly reports and an annual report sent to the MOHP. At the program level, it is not clear how the information on emerging patterns and trends in the region is shared with the GEIS Central Hub or with other GEIS sites, other than through publications in various international scientific journals and through annual reports.

### Conclusions

The IT environment at NAMRU-3 is sufficient to support the achievement of GEIS information objectives. The LISA system supports the NAMRU-3 GEIS priority of archiving selected specimens and epidemiological data for future investigations. This environment would benefit from an overall information plan, including the integration of information systems, and the development of systematic means of expeditiously communicating surveillance information to short- and long-term users (e.g., a NAMRU-3 website dedicated to surveillance).

## SURVEILLANCE

Surveillance activities were conducted by NAMRU-3 before the advent of GEIS. The GEIS focus on infectious diseases surveillance and response was added in fiscal year 1997 to the existing NAMRU-3 operating structure, which was historically dedicated to laboratory- and field-based infectious disease research. A GEIS implementation plan that takes advantage of existing projects has been developed for fiscal years 2000 to 2004. GEIS at NAMRU-3 is organized around five core areas or goals that include the following (GEIS, 1999a, 2000b; NAMRU-3, 2000a):

- enhanced surveillance for priority infectious diseases in Egypt;
- regional surveillance for selected diseases in Middle Eastern, Eastern European, Western Asian, and African countries;
- surveillance for infectious diseases in U.S. multinational forces and observers;
- surveillance and response to outbreaks in the WHO EMRO; and
- archiving of selected specimens and epidemiological data for future investigations.

These goals are linked to the priorities defined by the GEIS Central Hub in the following four pillar areas: influenza surveillance, drug-resistant malaria surveillance, surveillance for diseases caused by drug-resistant enteric pathogens, and acute febrile illness surveillance. The four RSD programs have worked together to define the activities described above. Their GEIS project applications and progress reports are submitted to the GEIS Central Hub on an annual basis.

### *Enhanced Surveillance for Priority Infectious Diseases in Egypt*

NAMRU-3 has developed protocols funded by GEIS to incorporate the pillars noted above. In particular, NAMRU-3 is developing a capacity for surveillance for a number of clinical syndromes including acute undifferentiated febrile illnesses, meningitis-encephalitis, viral hemorrhagic fevers, influenza, and dysentery. Since 1998, GEIS has supported projects to further develop efforts related to the surveillance of patients with meningitis-encephalitis in a network of infectious disease hospitals ("fever hospitals") in Egypt. Laboratory training and supplies have been provided in selected hospitals to upgrade clinical and microbiological capabilities. Clinical specimens are sent to NAMRU-3 for virological workups and other testing. Currently, surveillance is being conducted in 12 sites in 10 of 28 Egyptian governorates; and the scope of work has broadened to include patients with other in-country priority diseases such as typhoid fever, brucellosis, and viral hepatitis.

With GEIS funding, the Virology Research Program and the Disease Surveillance Program are working together to identify the causes of meningitis and encephalitis and to evaluate patients with acute febrile illness in selected governorates. The Enteric Diseases Research Program and the Disease Surveillance Program are collaborating on a project to implement surveillance for dysentery and severe diarrhea in selected populations. NAMRU-3 has also developed considerable capacity to conduct population-based surveillance (e.g., children with diarrhea in the Abu Homos field site and patients with acute fever of unknown origin in Upper Egypt).

NAMRU-3 has participated in a number of additional activities related to disease surveillance in Egypt. In 1998, the Egyptian MOHP formed a surveillance working group consisting of the MOHP Central Laboratory and the CDC Field Epidemiology Training Program (FETP), the WHO Regional Office, the U.S. Agency for International Development (USAID), and NAMRU-3. The primary goals and objectives of this working group were to develop a capacity for surveillance of infectious diseases in Egypt.

In 1999, the WHO Regional Office convened an expert panel to review the activities of existing communicable disease surveillance programs in Egypt (e.g., programs for the surveillance of polio, tuberculosis, and human immunodeficiency virus [HIV] infection/AIDS) and proposed an action plan to strengthen the national surveillance and response system. The expert panel, in which NAMRU-3 played a key role, made a number of recommendations regarding the strengthening of communicable disease surveillance in Egypt (NAMRU-3, 2000b). USAID and the government of Egypt are the primary providers of funding to support the implementation of the action plan advised by the panel. This allows NAMRU-3 to target funds from GEIS mainly toward regional surveillance and response activities, although GEIS remains essential in providing technical support in Egypt.

#### *Regional Surveillance for Selected Diseases in Middle Eastern, Eastern European, Western Asian, and African Countries*

A variety of surveillance-related projects are conducted in the region; in Egypt, Yemen, Syria, Djibouti, Turkey, Ghana, and Hungary, for instance. NAMRU-3 conducts focused surveillance and operational research activities in the region for influenza (Egypt and Syria and planned in

Djibouti), dengue (initiated in Djibouti and Yemen), and antimalarial drug resistance (planned in Yemen and Ghana).

*Surveillance for Infectious Diseases in Military Populations*

Serological studies of cohorts of U.S. multinational forces and observers (MFOs) in the Sinai have been and are still conducted by NAMRU-3. These studies have documented significant rates of incidence of West Nile encephalitis virus and sandfly fever virus infections. Surveillance for influenza among MFO troops is also conducted. In Turkey, a project has investigated gastroenteritis in locally deployed U.S. military personnel.

*Surveillance and Response to Outbreaks in the WHO EMRO*

See the section Response later in this chapter.

*Archiving of Selected Specimens and Epidemiological Data for Future Investigations*

See the section Technology and Information Management earlier in this chapter.

## Conclusions

In addition to infectious disease research in the field, NAMRU-3 activities now formally encompass infectious disease surveillance and response, including the provision of support for national public health infectious disease surveillance infrastructure. The introduction of GEIS has brought to NAMRU-3 a broader framework and additional resources. These resources allow NAMRU-3 to better assess and respond to infectious disease threats within the region in partnership with WHO and with relevant countries and relevant institutions. Establishing GEIS within the research framework of NAMRU-3 (funded by the Military Infectious Disease Research Program [MIDRP]) benefits both MIDRP and GEIS in a synergistic fashion: GEIS benefits from the scientific and technical facilities, staff expertise, established research efforts, and working relationships already in existence. In return, GEIS strengthens and builds partnerships and provides surveillance information useful to guide the development of future MIDRP-funded research projects, maximizing the benefits to the U.S. military as well as to Egypt and the surrounding region.

The GEIS framework and the links between projects that it provides have enhanced many NAMRU-3 research protocols. Although NAMRU-3 is successfully taking advantage of the skill and experience of its staff, as well as the technical and political opportunities available within the region, closer coordination of the various GEIS projects at NAMRU-3 and increased capacity in epidemiology would benefit GEIS.

Overall, NAMRU-3 is in a unique position to provide essential surveillance information related to infectious disease threats in Egypt and the region, including information on acute respiratory infections, arbovirus infections, viral hepatitis, and enteric diseases. Projects provide essential data regarding long-term trends in the antibiotic resistance of enteric pathogens and the incidence of diseases caused by arboviruses. Studies of military populations, together with information obtained from in-country and regional surveillance activities, work to provide a comprehensive picture of the potential infectious disease threats facing U.S. military forces. Regional infectious disease surveillance efforts also expand NAMRU-3's working relationships and partnerships within and outside of Egypt.

The subcommittee questions whether the current annual review and funding process allows sufficient time for surveillance project maturation and planning between reviews. Annual review appears to rush the proposal preparation process and can culminate in the making of decisions about the merits of projects on the basis of incomplete information.

## RESPONSE CAPACITY

Epidemics of known or emerging infectious diseases occur regularly in the region. Requests for assistance from the Egyptian MOHP or the WHO are directed to NAMRU-3's commanding officer, who determines the degree to which NAMRU-3 can assist. The mission of GEIS and the GEIS funding apparatus are used to facilitate timely responses to epidemics. NAMRU-3 can rapidly bring epidemiological and laboratory expertise to the field when epidemics occur and can also offer technical support to confirm diagnoses and to provide advice to the authorities that request it. NAMRU-3's administrative, medical, logistical, and scientific capabilities have all been called into play in assessing and managing epidemics in the region. In addition, the partnerships that NAMRU-3 has established with the Egyptian MOHP, other countries, and EMRO provide prompt clearances by the countries involved so that personnel and equipment can be brought to the field in a timely manner.

In recent years, NAMRU-3 has provided technical support to several epidemic investigations, including the following:

- acute gastroenteritis among U.S. Department of Defense (DoD) forces at Incirlik, Turkey, 1999;
- cluster of unexplained deaths among infants in Gharbia governorate, Egypt, 1999 (methanol intoxication);

• cluster of unexplained illness with skin lesions, Egypt, 2000 (accidental exposure to radiation);

• epidemic of Rift Valley fever in Yemen, 2000. The NAMRU-3 response to this epidemic was quite apparent at the time of the subcommittee visit to Cairo. The support provided by NAMRU-3 at the request of EMRO during this investigation included the establishment of a field laboratory in less than 1 week and the rapid design and implementation of an epidemiological investigation of both humans and animals. Importantly, this was the first report of Rift Valley fever outside Africa. NAMRU-3's unique capacity to rapidly investigate and respond to emerging infections in the region was clearly demonstrated, despite the tense political situation (related to the October attack on the USS *Cole* at Aden, Yemen). Although the investigators were from a U.S. military organization, they did not experience any significant security problems, undoubtedly because NAMRU-3 is primarily perceived in the region as a well-respected scientific institution rather than a military establishment.

### Conclusions

NAMRU-3's capabilities to respond to epidemics of potential public health or military significance are unsurpassed in the region in terms of laboratory diagnosis, field investigation, and collaboration (e.g., with the Egyptian MOHP and the WHO). The mission of GEIS and the GEIS funding apparatus have greatly facilitated timely responses to epidemics. The GEIS program has enhanced and strengthened the unique regional capacity of NAMRU-3. NAMRU-3 efforts in response to the Rift Valley fever epidemic were an impressive example of NAMRU-3's response capability.

## COLLABORATIONS

Public health partners are receiving NAMRU-3 support in the following areas:

• isolation and identification of "exotic" or emerging viruses in the region;

• rapid deployment of field diagnostic capacity in support of outbreak investigations;

• production of diagnostic reagents (e.g., specific antigens) not commercially available;

• collection, transportation, and storage of vast quantities and varieties of clinical specimens, including maintenance of a unique regional serum bank; and

• strengthening of the overall laboratory capacity in the region, particularly in Egypt, through training and quality control programs, usually associated with specific NAMRU-3 research or surveillance projects.

NAMRU-3 has many partners, including the Egyptian MOHP, governmental agencies of other countries in the region, other DoD departments, and a range of technical and financial partners such as the WHO, the CDC, and USAID. Partner agencies visited by the subcommittee spoke highly of the work and responsiveness of the laboratory and offered strong support for NAMRU-3's activities. The subcommittee also heard from staff at NAMRU-3 and from NAMRU-3's partners that the introduction of GEIS has expanded NAMRU-3's mandate and range of partners. Before GEIS, NAMRU-3 had no explicit mission to strengthen the capacity of the MOHP. Joint planning and programming are well established with the MOHP. Within the MOHP, key partners include the FETP, the Central Laboratory, the fever hospitals, and field sites such as those that the subcommittee visited in Abu Homos.

Staff and partners alike reported being very pleased at the development of GEIS, noting that it had increased the relevance of the work of the laboratory both to the country and to the surrounding region. The U.S. Embassy's deputy chief of mission praised the work of NAMRU-3 in Egypt, noting that the NAMRU-3 partnership with the MOHP takes many forms, including training and staff development and the provision of equipment and supplies for laboratory-based surveillance efforts, most of which are being funded by USAID. In all visits to MOHP facilities, concern was expressed about the need for and the sustainability of a strong surveillance effort for infectious diseases and the need for the Egyptian MOHP to accept responsibility for maintaining and expanding the current surveillance activities. NAMRU-3 staff also mentioned that input from experts (a review team or similar source) regarding the development of Egyptian public health laboratory capacity and surveillance activities would be useful and might be something that GEIS could help procure.

NAMRU-3 also has collaborative relationships with other countries under EMRO's purview, such as Yemen, Sudan, Djibouti, and Turkey. The EMRO director of communicable diseases also spoke highly of NAMRU-3 and its proactive approach to strengthening the surveillance and response systems within the region. NAMRU-3 is a WHO Collaborating Center for HIV, for cholera, and for emerging infectious diseases. Among financial partners, the USAID mission in Egypt also praised the work and approach of NAMRU-3 and reported confidence in expanding its partnership with NAMRU-3 to implement key surveillance-related projects in Egypt. Information sharing relationships between NAMRU-3 and its partners appear strong, but seem person-based and circumstance dependent.

The assignment of a CDC public health professional to NAMRU-3 makes CDC a key technical partner of NAMRU-3. Other DoD entities, such as the U.S. Army Medical Research Institute of Infectious Diseases and other military laboratories operating overseas, are also essential partners with NAMRU-3. However, it was not completely clear to the IOM subcommittee how communication and coordination with the GEIS Central Hub and other GEIS sites is realized.

### Conclusions

NAMRU-3 has been very successful in developing and maintaining a range of local, national, regional, and international partnerships. In particular, the GEIS mission has increased the possibilities for capacity building with the Egyptian MOHP in support of improved surveillance and response. NAMRU-3 support to the Central Laboratory, enhanced by GEIS, has been crucial in the last few years in building new laboratory capacity in Egypt. GEIS could also provide supervision for the training of in-country laboratory workers for a limited time to improve communicable disease surveillance in the country. This training will, in turn, support the GEIS mission at NAMRU-3. It is important that the capacity-building efforts of NAMRU-3 be directed to the development of systems that can be sustained by the Egyptian government.

The level of appreciation and confidence expressed by partners regarding NAMRU-3 were noteworthy. NAMRU-3 is viewed by its various stakeholders as an asset for infectious disease research in the field and is deemed important to the region. GEIS is now seen as a means of applying some of the pertinent research and surveillance findings to public health practice in Egypt and in the surrounding region. GEIS at NAMRU-3 thus serves as a cornerstone for the promotion of infectious disease surveillance in the region. This positions NAMRU-3 well for the development of new partnerships, including those needed to generate additional financial and political resources.

It should be acknowledged that these successful partnership may sometimes bring competing priorities to the table. These competing priorities can be dealt with only by reiterating and promoting the GEIS core surveillance goals to these partners at every opportunity.

## RECOMMENDATIONS

- GEIS activities at NAMRU-3 are of critical importance to the program as a whole. The committee encourages the DoD to plan for GEIS activities at NAMRU-3 on a long-term basis. NAMRU-3 provides an important resource for both research and surveillance missions. Demand for and support of these missions should be balanced so that neither one is jeopardized.

**Recommendation: DoD commitment to GEIS at NAMRU-3 should be long term.**

• The current annual approval process does not allow optimal time for NAMRU-3 project planning or maturation. Furthermore, it is important that the GEIS Central Hub review and approval process for GEIS projects provides NAMRU-3 with follow-up guidance regarding project progress in a consistent and timely manner (see also Chapter 7).

**Recommendation: Consideration should be given to revising the current GEIS project application and review process.**

• The assignment of additional civilian epidemiologists (from CDC and other relevant institutions) or the assignment of DoD epidemiologists or public health specialists to NAMRU-3 is essential to fulfill GEIS objectives. Improved communication by the GEIS Central Hub of the mission of GEIS to NAMRU-3 is also needed. Providing existing staff with additional training in epidemiology, public health, and public health surveillance could also help meet the need for additional applied epidemiology expertise at NAMRU-3.

**Recommendation: Additional applied epidemiological input should be provided to guide the development and conduct of NAMRU-3 GEIS projects to fully realize program goals.**

**Recommendation: Consideration should be given to obtaining a full-time, on-site manager possessing experience in applied epidemiology and public health for the GEIS program at NAMRU-3, or to providing more epidemiological and technical oversight responsibility to the manager of the Disease Surveillance Program, as the current NAMRU-3 organizational structure does not allow the Disease Surveillance Program to maximize collaboration and coordination of GEIS activities across the Research Sciences Department.**

• FSN staff can help meet staffing needs in areas, such as epidemiology, for which there is presently a shortage of qualified DoD personnel. FSNs also help to provide continuity between projects and in relationships with partner agencies.

**Recommendation: NAMRU-3 should ensure the long-term presence of FSN personnel to maximize the continuity of individual GEIS projects and provide the institutional memory and cultural sensitivity necessary for the success of GEIS.**

• NAMRU-3 has been very successful in developing and maintaining a range of local, national, regional, and international partnerships.

**Recommendation: NAMRU-3, in coordination with the GEIS Central Hub, should expand partnerships with and continue to raise funds through (as applicable) sources such as USAID (country offices and its Global Bureau), the CDC (including the FETP), the WHO, and other relevant agencies to the full extent possible to enhance in-country surveillance and response capacities.**

**Recommendation: NAMRU-3 should continue to support the Egyptian MOHP in gradually strengthening the MOHP's own capacity for surveillance across Egypt, with a particular focus on laboratory diagnostic capabilities. This support should also be extended to other countries in the region, resources permitting.**

- The sharing of information with partners in public health activities, particularly those positioned to take action in response to epidemics, should be timely and systematic.

**Recommendation: A comprehensive NAMRU-3 information plan that outlines the needs and mechanisms for the reporting of information to partners in public health activities and to the GEIS Central Hub should be developed and acted upon.**

**Recommendation: NAMRU-3 should actively pursue with its in-country partners resolution of issues regarding ownership of surveillance data and issues regarding the clearance of data for dissemination.**

- The subcommittee recognizes that the GEIS pillar disease areas are important ones and that defining these targets helps to provide some standardization of GEIS activities across sites, but the pillar structure should be flexible enough to permit, on a case-by-case basis, local infectious diseases that are of global concern (e.g., tuberculosis) to be addressed as high priorities through GEIS. This serves to take full advantage of the epidemiological setting of the facility, builds national health defenses in the host country, and can be of long-term benefit to the health of many populations, including U.S. military personnel and civilians.

**Recommendation: Consideration should be given to refining the focus of GEIS at NAMRU-3 to better enable diseases outside of the pillar areas to be addressed.**

- Partnerships benefit from knowledge of the native language by senior staff. Partnerships are of increased importance to NAMRU-3 now that its research mission has been formally expanded to include GEIS activities, which necessitate increased interactions with partner agencies.

Staff familiarity and comfort with the local language can also improve rates of retention of personnel and assist in cultural acclimation.

**Recommendation: Senior staff at NAMRU-3 actively involved in GEIS projects should be conversant in the dominant language of the host country or should be encouraged to pursue, with the support of GEIS, language training, and should seek to become conversant to the extent possible.**

## PEOPLE MET AND INTERVIEWED

### *NAMRU-3 Staff*

Edward Antosek
Cole Church
Elizabeth A. Dykstra
Robert W. Frenck, Jr.
Ross Graham
Frank J. Mahoney
James Malone
Moustafa M. Mansour

### *NAMRU-3 Associates*

Heda Mansour, Abassia Fever Hospital
Mark Anthony White, USAID
Deputy Chief of Mission, U.S. Embassy
Dr. Zoheir Halaj, WHO representative, Egypt
Dr. Nasser, director, FETP Egypt

## ITINERARY

### *October 8*

| | |
|---|---|
| 0900–0930 | Command brief |
| 0930–1000 | GEIS project overview |
| 1000–1100 | Disease surveillance program brief and tour |
| 1100–1130 | Enteric disease research program brief and tour |
| 1130–1300 | Lunch |
| 1300–1400 | Virology research program brief and tour |
| 1400–1430 | Vector biology research program brief and tour |

***October 9***

| | |
|---|---|
| 0840–1300 | Meetings:<br>Central laboratory, Ministry of Health and Population<br>World Health Organization, Country Representative Office<br>Field Epidemiology Training Program<br>Ministry of Health<br>Eastern Mediterranean Regional Office, World Health Organization<br>Deputy Chief of Mission, U.S. Embassy |

***October 10***

| | |
|---|---|
| 0840 | Meetings with USAID personnel |

***October 11***

| | |
|---|---|
| | *K. Gensheimer and J. Hospedales* |
| 0730 | Depart hotel for Alexandria |
| 0930–1030 | Mahalla El-Kobra Fever Hospital |
| 1200–1500 | Abu Homos Clinic brief and site visit |
| | *G. Rodier* |
| 0500 | Depart hotel for Luxor |
| 1030 | Quena fever hospital (canceled for security reasons) |
| 1300 | Cohort study |

***October 12***

| | |
|---|---|
| | *K. Gensheimer and J. Hospedales* |
| 0900 | Alexandria Fever Hospital |
| | *G. Rodier* |
| 0900 | Armunt Fever Hospital (done under military escort) |

***October 13***

| | |
|---|---|
| | Follow-up discussion with NAMRU-3 staff<br>Writing of subcommittee report |

***October 14***

| | |
|---|---|
| | Depart for Kenya |

# 6

# GEIS at U.S. Army Medical Research Unit, Kenya

The U.S. Army Medical Research Unit, Kenya (USAMRU-K), was first established in 1969 as a temporary program put in place at the invitation of the Kenyan government to study trypanosomiasis. In 1973, USAMRU-K was made permanent through a cooperative agreement between the Walter Reed Army Institute of Research (WRAIR), Washington, D.C., and the Kenya Medical Research Institute (KEMRI), the Kenyan governmental agency responsible for all biomedical research in Kenya. Research focused on the immunobiology of trypanosomiasis and on the development of a potential vaccine until the early 1980s, when investigators began research on Rift Valley fever, malaria epidemiology, and clinical and field aspects of leishmaniasis. USAMRU-K operates as a WRAIR Special Foreign Activity and is unofficially known within Kenya as "The Walter Reed Project" (Gambel and Hibbs, 1996; GEIS, 2001f).

USAMRU-K has worked primarily as a research organization since its inception. Historically, USAMRU-K has been dedicated to and supported by applied medical research, and its charter and invitation to operate in Kenya are founded on its research mission. Approximately $500,000 was received from GEIS during fiscal year 2000 (USAMRU-K, 2000). In fiscal year 2001, GEIS is expected to supply USAMRU-K with approximately $460,000 (GEIS, 2000c). The majority of USAMRU-K's budget, which amounted to $2.5 million in 2000, comes from the U.S. Military Infectious Diseases Research Program (MIDRP). Congressional appropriations for a human immunodeficiency virus (HIV) vaccine and prevention of HIV infection/AIDS, the Intra-Laboratory Innovative Research program of the U.S. Department of Defense (DoD), and various grants and subsidies from commercial partners and granting agencies also support USAMRU-K.

To date, the principal activities of USAMRU-K have included the following:

- Investigation of basic immune responses to the malaria parasite and HIV;
- testing of drugs against the malaria parasite and HIV and testing of antimalarial drugs and drug resistance;
- development and testing of simplified diagnostics for malaria, leishmaniasis, and dengue;
- epidemiology and control of vector-borne diseases; and
- epidemic response (e.g., Rift Valley fever and Marburg virus infection).

A subcommittee of the Institute of Medicine (IOM) Committee to Review the Department of Defense Global Emerging Infections Surveillance and Response System visited USAMRU-K from October 16 to 20, 2000. The subcommittee consisted of committee members Kathleen Gensheimer, James Hospedales, and Guénaël Rodier. G. Rodier was recalled on October 17 to coordinate the World Health Organization (WHO) response to an epidemic of viral hemorrhagic fever in Uganda. A list of the people met and the itinerary followed can be found at the end of this chapter.

## LABORATORY

In 1985, KEMRI took occupancy of new laboratory facilities in Nairobi, and USAMRU-K headquarters were moved into this new KEMRI space. Research teams from the U.S. Centers for Disease Control and Prevention (CDC) and the Japanese International Cooperation Agency (JICA) are also collocated on the KEMRI campus.

In Nairobi, USAMRU-K headquarters are housed within the KEMRI Clinical Research Center, 1 of 10 KEMRI centers. In addition to a floor of laboratories and offices that house bacteriology, entomology, parasitology, and molecular biology activities at USAMRU-K headquarters in Nairobi, field operations are maintained at the western location of Kisian on Lake Victoria (for malaria studies) and at the high-elevation site of Kericho (for HIV studies). Smaller sites are maintained at Kisii in the highlands (for cerebral malaria), Baringo in the Rift Valley (for leishmaniasis), and Kilifi on the coast (for dengue). Limited virological capabilities are available within KEMRI through the KEMRI Center for Virus Research, a WHO Collaborating Center for Arbovirus and Viral Hemorrhagic Fever Reference and Research. This laboratory is not directly administered by USAMRU-K, although Global Emerging Infections Surveillance and Response System (GEIS) resources are contributed to support it. The KEMRI Center for Virus Research also receives support, through a series of complex arrangements, from other agencies such as the CDC and the WHO. At the time of the subcommittee's visit, the KEMRI Center for Virus Research did not possess the technology and reagents necessary to diagnose Ebola, Marburg, Lassa, or Crimean-Congo hemorrhagic fever.[1] The U.S. Army Medical Research Institute of Infectious Diseases does not routinely provide USAMRU-K with reagents or supplies (Ludwig, 2001).

Boundaries between those operations and facilities that are specific to KEMRI and those that belong to USAMRU-K are difficult to discern. Some laboratory space is occupied solely by USAMRU-K or by KEMRI, and other space (such as facilities for the detection and evaluation of enteric pathogens) is shared. In shared laboratories, USAMRU-K supplies many reagents, supplies, and equipment for common use. USAMRU-K facilities operate at a biosafety level 2 capacity, though biosafety level 3 capabilities are available through the KEMRI Center for Virus Research.

Much of USAMRU-K's work is conducted at field sites (USAMRU-K, 2000). Although the subcommittee did not visit the site, the field laboratory in Kisian (shared with the KEMRI Center for Vector Biology and Control Research) reportedly exceeded its operating capacity years ago. Several current field activities, such as global positioning system work and drug studies, have had to set up in hotel and rented quarters. Plans exist to build a new facility at this site. GEIS funds may be used to equip the facility.

USAMRU-K operations are substantially affected by infrastructure limitations in the country. Basic functionalities that are generally taken for granted in developed countries, such as electrical power, can be in short supply because of frequent power outages and rationing. Two freezers (purchased with GEIS funds) for the storage of specimens for drug testing have yet to be plugged in because no outlets are available. Emergency power is undependable and inadequate. Communications within and outside of the country are likewise erratic, as even the most basic technological support, such as a telephone system, is not always available (USAMRU-K, 2000). Also, operations in Kenya take a relatively harsh toll on equipment. For instance, because of hazardous road conditions and theft, the effective lives of all motor vehicles in Kenya are less than 5 years.

[1]Steps are being taken to make these reagents regularly available to KEMRI (Dunster, 2001; Ludwig, 2001).

### Conclusions

The location of USAMRU-K in Kenya, a country that is geographically diverse and rich in transmissible pathogens, offers exciting potential for the study of emerging infectious diseases in country as well as within the region. Kenya's troubled infrastructure gives rise to operational challenges and, at the same time, heightens the need for GEIS efforts. To achieve program objectives, investment in improving national public health capacity is crucial. Continued investment in improving USAMRU-K's laboratory capabilities is a part of this process.

At all sites that the IOM subcommittee visited, USAMRU-K's physical facilities range from marginally adequate to basic. In addition, lack of reagents such as those that would be necessary to enable capabilities for the diagnosis of viral hemorrhagic fevers limits USAMRU-K's capacity to achieve its full potential as part of GEIS.

## STAFFING

The U.S. Army authorizes USAMRU-K a contingent of nine professional and two administrative U.S. personnel. Despite adequate funding, only five Army officers and one GS-11 civilian were assigned to the unit at the time of the subcommittee's visit. In addition to the U.S. staff, USAMRU-K employs about 120 Kenyan technical staff through a contractual agreement with KEMRI. Nonmilitary USAMRU-K personnel are actually contracted to KEMRI through annually renewable contracts. There is currently no doctoral-level Kenyan national on staff at USAMRU-K, although arrangements are in place to have a physician assigned to USAMRU-K from KEMRI's Center for Clinical Research. This physician is to work in association with a preventive medicine officer to be posted at USAMRU-K later in 2001. This preventive medicine officer is to work full time on GEIS activities.

The lack of a virologist among USAMRU-K staff assignees was noted. Although USAMRU-K can use the services of the KEMRI virologist, this individual is primarily responsible to KEMRI and other institutes of the Kenyan Ministry of Health (MoH). At the time of the site visit, this individual was heavily engaged with the MoH, attempting to provide public health-type advice regarding the establishment of a surveillance system for Ebola virus in Kenya, and was unavailable to provide virological support for ongoing activities or for diagnostic responses. Additional virological support could have made USAMRU-K a key player in the Ebola virus epidemic. The salaries of three technicians who work with the KEMRI virologist and most of the supplies used by the virologist in his work are paid for directly by USAMRU-K with GEIS funds.

As an aside, the efforts of USAMRU-K staff to learn Swahili are noteworthy, as such skills help to integrate projects and foster collaborative associations with the public health community in the host country.

## Conclusions

A net loss of personnel, including the loss of three of four medical officers, during the 18 months leading up to the subcommittee's site visit has made it difficult for USAMRU-K to achieve its objectives. This loss of personnel has interfered with GEIS implementation. The subcommittee recognizes that USAMRU-K is obligated to all agencies (chiefly MIDRP) and partners from which it accepts funds and that juggling such responsibilities presents a challenge to a laboratory that is understaffed, underscoring the need to recruit and retain competent staff.

USAMRU-K is particularly deficient in staff who possess expertise in public health and epidemiology and who can be available on site to guide USAMRU-K as it moves beyond its traditional research-based mission to substantially and substantively support public health-focused activities as well. Although a U.S. Army physician-epidemiologist is scheduled to join USAMRU-K in September 2001, other staffing options also warrant consideration. Additional senior-level foreign service nationals could offer further public health and epidemiological expertise, as well as insight into the working of the country. The current lack of foreign service nationals among senior-level staff at USAMRU-K represents a missed opportunity for USAMRU-K and for GEIS. Given the scope of GEIS and the threat that viral infectious disease entities pose in Kenya and the region, the placement of another virologist within the KEMRI laboratory, funded by USAMRU-K, may also be worth considering for the purposes of expanding the scope of virological surveillance activities in country and providing USAMRU-K and GEIS with better access to virological support. GEIS at USAMRU-K would also benefit from a full-time, on-site manager, possessing applied epidemiology and public health expertise.

Efforts to become integrated with the culture of the host country work well to enhance working relationships and help stimulate research and surveillance activities. The presence of native-born professionals, such as the senior research officer at the Center for Microbiology Research (KEMRI), actively working with GEIS significantly expands the scope of the in-country activities of USAMRU-K by providing cultural and linguistic links to government- and institution-based professionals within the country. Staff efforts to learn and communicate with collaborators in the local language similarly serve to enhance working relationships. The efforts of current U.S. military staff to learn Swahili are commendable.

## TECHNOLOGY AND INFORMATION MANAGEMENT

A range of information and communication technology resources are available within the KEMRI complex. Some have been recently acquired, in whole or in part, through GEIS. For example, a very-small-aperture-terminal (VSAT) system[2] installed 6 months before the site visit has greatly improved access to the Internet, facilitating e-mail communication, medical literature searches, and the sharing of data from field sites. The VSAT system supports satellite communications for USAMRU-K and its partners: CDC, JICA, WHO, and the Oxford-Wellcome Foundation. This KEMRI system is linked to the Multilateral Initiative on Malaria Communications Network (MIMCom) network,[3] which seeks to foster communication among malaria researchers in Africa (MIMCom, 2001) as part of a joint effort supported by the Fogarty Foundation and the National Library of Medicine of the U.S. National Institutes of Health (GEIS, 2000b). The director of KEMRI spoke highly of the value added by the VSAT system in a country where regular telephone communications are unreliable. He was also enthusiastic about the four computers recently purchased with GEIS funds and installed in KEMRI's library. A newly hired systems administrator has contributed to the improvement of the information technology infrastructure and is planning to introduce a KEMRI website, Voice Over Internet Protocol (VOIP), and an intranet. A local area network exists and is being upgraded.

However, an overall information plan—a comprehensive strategy for making use of technical resources to share information with and receive information from public health partners—does not exist. No regular surveillance bulletin or other means of routine distribution of GEIS project data is undertaken specifically by USAMRU-K, although KEMRI has plans to begin producing a quarterly newsletter that will provide updates on specimen numbers, diagnoses, epidemics, profiles of laboratory methods, staff profiles, and a forum for discussion. The commander of USAMRU-K acknowledged that the communication and sharing of information on disease patterns and trends with those who need to take action was an area in great need of improvement. Nor was it clear that information on emerging patterns and trends is shared with the GEIS Central Hub or other GEIS sites on a routine and timely basis. The commander of USAMRU-K expressed concern that guidance regarding dissemination of

---

[2]A VSAT receives information from and transmits to information terminals that have been installed at dispersed sites and that are connected to a central hub by satellite with small-diameter (0.6- to 3.8-meter) antenna dishes (Spread Spectrum Scene Online, 2001).

[3]In Nairobi, the communications infrastructure is supplied by USAMRU-K; in western Kenya, MIMCom and the National Library of Medicine supply this infrastructure.

GEIS surveillance data and planning for dissemination of GEIS surveillance data have been insufficient.

USAMRU-K does not yet have a laboratory information system to facilitate laboratory management and surveillance needs.

### Conclusions

The information technology environment at USAMRU-K is sufficient, despite infrastructure challenges in Kenya, to support the achievement of GEIS objectives. The VSAT system—and the communications support that it provides—represents a valuable investment by GEIS.

GEIS at USAMRU-K would benefit from the development of an overall information plan, including the development of a laboratory information system, and the development of systematic means of communicating surveillance information to short- and long-term data users, including the MoH as well as other GEIS sites.

## SURVEILLANCE

USAMRU-K conducted several surveillance-related activities before the introduction of GEIS, although it cannot be said that an applied public health surveillance program was in place. The GEIS focus on infectious disease surveillance and response was added in fiscal year 1997 to the existing USAMRU-K operating structure, historically dedicated to laboratory-based infectious disease research.

A GEIS implementation plan for fiscal years 2000 through 2004 has been developed. The primary areas of USAMRU-K GEIS program focus are as follows:

- strengthening of the infrastructure for surveillance,
- surveillance for the agents of dysentery and associated antibiotic resistance,
- surveys of hantavirus and rickettsia in Kenya,
- surveillance for viral hemorrhagic fevers, and
- surveillance for drug resistance in malaria parasites.

*Infrastructure Strengthening*

The infrastructure for surveillance and communication in Kenya is poor. Information technology capabilities within the MoH appear to be very limited for effective disease surveillance and information sharing. MoH capabilities are heavily dependent on the resources of its collaborators.

One of the first GEIS undertakings has been the installation of a VSAT system dish and related communication technology at KEMRI (discussed in the section Technology and Information Management of this chapter). These efforts have increased the capacity for data management and information sharing. The installation of a backup generator at the KEMRI Virus Research Center has also contributed to strengthening of the infrastructure. Future plans include the expansion of the KEMRI communications network to connect all KEMRI investigators to the VSAT system and the contribution of funds to develop a laboratory with rooms dedicated to GEIS and geographic information system (GIS) work in Kisian. Other partners are also working to build the MoH's capacity; for instance, the WHO-supported project on integrated disease surveillance that started in 2000 has provided four computers and training to 4 of 10 Kenyan health districts involved in the project.

*Surveillance for Agents of Dysentery*

In a collaboration between USAMRU-K and the African Medical and Research Foundation (AMREF) and KEMRI, surveillance for agents of dysentery has commenced at Magadi-Entasopia, a site in southern Kenya near the border with Tanzania. This effort focuses on the Masai people, who live in or migrate through the area and who live in close proximity to livestock. AMREF has provided the study site, supplied initial coordination and guidance to clinic staff, and is supposed to analyze stool samples for parasites. KEMRI and USAMRU-K are primarily responsible for bacteriological analysis, antimicrobial susceptibility testing, and molecular and toxin characterization of isolates. However, USAMRU-K has not received information regarding parasitic analyses from AMREF since March 2000, when the study began. This surveillance project has shown that the most common causes of dysentery are enterotoxigenic *Escherichia coli* and *Shigella* and that multiple drug resistance is common among these organisms. This project has also resulted in the description of the first cases of verotoxic *Shigella flexneri, Shigella dysenteriae* type 12, and *E. coli* O157:H7 in Africa. Future work is to include an enterhemorrhagic *E. coli* study in slaughterhouses, slum districts, and rotating sites in Kenya and Eastern Africa. Renewal of the contract with AMREF and the conduct of active and passive surveillance at a number of clinics in Kenya and Eastern Africa are also planned. USAMRU-K reportedly intends to expand its work with enteric pathogens throughout the region to make use of the extensive network of Médicins Sans Frontières (MSF; Doctors Without Borders), an international medical aid organization that operates in Kenya and other countries in the region.

*Surveys of Hantavirus and Rickettsia*

Surveys of hantavirus and rickettsia have been conducted in collaboration with the WHO. Projects use the existing WHO Yellow Fever Surveillance Network. The hantavirus study is based in 24 mission and district hospitals in eight of the nine Kenyan provinces. Samples collected from patients with fever of unknown origin are tested. One of the study sites reported clinical presentations consistent with hantavirus infection, and serological evidence of infection was found in test sera. The study of rickettsial infection has just begun and is based on the collection of ticks from slaughterhouses and field sites around Kijabe Mission Hospital. It uses polymerase chain reaction techniques to provide evidence of infection. Tick bites of humans and livestock are a common occurrence, and several clinical cases suggestive of rickettsial infection were found. The patients responded to treatment with doxycycline. Future work on hantavirus is to include trapping and testing of rodents, expansion of the study to other locations, and analysis of possible arthropod vectors within the vector population. Future work on *Rickettsia* is to focus on suspected human cases by using serological surveys and on vector studies.

*Surveillance for Fevers of Unknown Origin and Viral Hemorrhagic Diseases*

Surveillance for fevers of unknown origin and viral hemorrhagic diseases is being undertaken in collaboration with the KEMRI Center for Virus Research and is based in the same 24 mission and district hospitals as the study of *Rickettsia*. The KEMRI virologist has been proactive in reactivating these sites for the purpose of limited surveillance for hemorrhagic fever, an effort that receives GEIS support. The subcommittee attended one of the sensitization sessions for this project at the Kijabe Mission Hospital in the Rift Valley. Future plans for work in this area include screening of specimens sent through the network for a range of possible causes of fever of unknown origin, including hantavirus and viral hemorrhagic fever. This work resulted in the discovery of endemic dengue transmission in coastal Kenya (GEIS, 2000b). Follow-up epidemiological investigations regarding dengue virus transmission are also intended to elucidate patterns of transmission and vector distribution.

*Surveillance for Drug Resistance in Malaria Parasites*

GEIS-funded studies for surveillance for drug resistance in malaria parasites have been conducted at Kericho and Kisumu, Nairobi, and Entasopia in west, central, and southern Kenya, respectively. Work involves comparison of the results of in vitro drug susceptibility testing with those of molecular biology-based analyses (polymerase chain reaction) for markers of resistance. Initial study results have shown very high levels of chloroquine resistance among malaria parasites and a positive correlation of that resistance with molecular markers. Future work is to include a retrospective 10-year study of mutation patterns, the development of laboratory capabilities, the provision of reference testing, and the development of a malaria parasite resistance database for East Africa.

*Other Surveillance Activities and Plans*

USAMRU-K has provided research training for many DoD preventive medicine residents and other scientists and students over the years. USAMRU-K has supported at least one trainee as part of the GEIS Overseas Medical Research Laboratory Orientation Training Program. As part of GEIS implementation, USAMRU-K has also developed a plan to coordinate epidemiology and epidemic response training for Kenyan nationals using University of Nairobi staff (USAMRU-K, 2000). This plan has not yet been implemented. USAMRU-K is not involved in the development of a new epidemiology training course that is to be offered in Kenya under the direction of the GEIS Central Hub and AMREF (McCarthy, 2000). The GEIS Central Hub, however, did not actively seek USAMRU-K involvement in this activity.

Plans also exist to develop methods that can be used to predict atypical patterns of transmission of important pathogens, especially those that are vector borne. Focus will be on identifying patterns resulting from environmental changes. This venture will be undertaken in partnership with the International Livestock Research Institute (ILRI), which, as noted above, has an impressive GIS capability.

## Conclusions

USAMRU-K is well positioned to meet the goals and objectives of GEIS and can substantially contribute to a global infectious disease surveillance and response network. Current and planned surveillance activities are generally in line with the GEIS mission, but these activities could be expanded, resources permitting. Also, present USAMRU-K GEIS activities appear to represent a collection of individual projects rather than respective parts of a cohesive program. GEIS at USAMRU-K would benefit from better integration of the projects.

Establishment of GEIS within the research framework of USAMRU-K (USAMRU-K research activities are funded primarily by MIDRP) can benefit both MIDRP and GEIS in a synergistic fashion: GEIS can benefit from the scientific and technical facilities, staff expertise, established research efforts, and working relationships already in existence. In return, GEIS can strengthen and build partnerships and can provide surveillance information useful in guiding the development of future MIDRP-funded research projects that maximize benefits to the U.S. military, as well as to Kenya and the surrounding region. Finding a balance between these missions is important to the success of both and to the effective functioning of USAMRU-K.

Expansion of key partnerships such as those with the MoH and the WHO can greatly increase the success of USAMRU-K GEIS activities. Provision of training in epidemiology, as planned, would also help to build the competences and capacities necessary to support emerging infectious disease surveillance in Kenya. These training activities seem supportive of the MoH plans and the WHO project, but USAMRU-K must be a leader in all GEIS efforts in the region—including but not limited to training.

The Geographic Information System (GIS) activities being developed in collaboration with ILRI have much potential to enhance surveillance for emerging infectious diseases. However, as all surveillance data need to result in information for action, it is important to develop a plan for transmission of this information to the MoH in such a way that it will be useful for response at the national, district, and local levels. For instance, combining the human vector information with information from expanded veterinary epidemiological activities could enhance surveillance and response activities for emerging zoonotic diseases.

Influenza is not considered a priority disease in Kenya, and to date, it has not been a part of GEIS efforts there. However, because influenza is one of the GEIS pillars and because influenza surveillance activities are lacking throughout much of Africa, it would be prudent to capture some information regarding currently circulating influenza viruses to enhance the global influenza surveillance effort.

## RESPONSE CAPACITY

Epidemics of emerging infectious diseases with known and unknown origins occur regularly in Kenya and within Eastern Africa. The MoH is currently involved in pulling together resources to implement for Kenya a plan of action for the management of disease epidemics. The plan attempts to outline the resources required to respond to the priority diseases in the country. The MoH is seeking to establish rapid response teams to deal with crisis infectious disease situations.

During the subcommittee site visit to USAMRU-K, an epidemic of Ebola virus was occurring in neighboring Uganda. USAMRU-K was only an observer of the response team assembled to deal with the crisis. Although the MoH spent a great deal of effort attempting to prevent importation of the virus into Kenya and dedicated epidemic response teams to border locations to create surveillance sites for the virus, the role of

USAMRU-K remained limited. Although Kenya is geographically situated in a region of Africa that has experienced repeated epidemics of viral hemorrhagic fever, and despite repeated requests to the international scientific community for the appropriate reagents for the diagnosis of Ebola, Lassa, and Marburg fevers, such reagents have not been regularly made available to the KEMRI Center for Virus Research, which USAMRU-K relies upon for virology diagnostic capabilities.

In 1997–1998, during a Rift Valley fever epidemic in Kenya, USAMRU-K was reportedly active in epidemic response efforts. It was also reported that at the time of this epidemic, additional diagnostic tools and staff resources were available to USAMRU-K.

## Conclusions

Emerging infectious disease response is one of the goals of GEIS outlined in the GEIS strategic plan (GEIS, 1998). One objective of GEIS is to "establish mechanisms and partnerships needed to ensure rapid and effective development and implementation of assessment, response, and prevention measures" (GEIS, 1998, p. 36). At present, USAMRU-K is not in a position to accomplish this objective.

To optimize response capacity, USAMRU-K needs to work with the MoH and other partners to enhance the surveillance system within Kenya so that epidemics can be detected and reported to the MoH in a timely fashion. Without this capacity for surveillance, epidemics may never be detected or reported to the central government. Until USAMRU-K becomes fully integrated with other potential partners, USAMRU-K will remain on the sidelines as an observer rather than being called in as an active participant.

USAMRU-K needs to be a fully staffed and equipped facility if it is to provide adequate support in an epidemic situation. USAMRU-K needs to have the technical, professional, and laboratory capacities required to provide assistance in response to requests from the MoH, the WHO, or other sub-Saharan African countries. Such requests may be for assistance with the identification of an etiological agent and its mode of transmission or assistance with the implementation of the preventive strategies needed to end the epidemic. If capabilities for the rapid diagnosis of infectious disease entities that pose a significant public health threat and sufficient applied epidemiological expertise are not consistently made available to USAMRU-K, the laboratory will not be in an optimal position to be a full partner in responding to disease entities that exist on its doorstep.

## COLLABORATIONS

KEMRI is a component of the MoH. Until recently, KEMRI operated under the direction of the Ministry of Education, Research, and Technology. KEMRI has 10 centers that report to a deputy director of research and development. As noted previously, USAMRU-K headquarters are physically located on the KEMRI campus in Nairobi, an arrangement that permits close collaborations with KEMRI scientists and other staff. USAMRU-K projects are integrated throughout KEMRI. For instance, USAMRU-K has collaborated with the Center for Microbiology Research on enteric disease and drug resistance studies. USAMRU-K and the Center for Virus Research have worked closely together to study such disease entities as arboviruses (the agent of yellow fever) and viral hemorrhagic fevers. Other collaborative projects have included work on dengue virus transmission, measles virus shedding in HIV-positive individuals, and a study of fevers of unknown origin. Since USAMRU-K moved into KEMRI space, KEMRI has administered all civilian personnel and has provided laboratory space, utilities, and vehicles as part of a renewable 3-year cooperative agreement. The arrangements for USAMRU-K collaborations with KEMRI centers are not governed by a cooperative agreement but are informally approved by the director of KEMRI.

The potential for collaborative relationships with other areas of the MoH also exists. The current head of the Division of Communicable Diseases (not part of KEMRI) indicated an interest in working with USAMRU-K. She specifically indicated an interest in involving USAMRU-K in setting up and facilitating the disease epidemic management units within Kenya; preparing and responding to disease epidemics; developing an integrated disease surveillance pilot project in collaboration with the WHO; and planning, implementing, and evaluating malaria control activities, an MoH priority. The MoH is currently involved in pulling together resources to implement for Kenya a plan of action for the management of disease epidemics. The plan attempts to outline the resources and response needs for priority diseases in the country, including cholera, bacillary dysentery, plague, measles, yellow fever, meningococcal meningitis, viral hemorrhagic fever, poliomyelitis, guinea worm infection, neonatal tetanus, leprosy, HIV infection, tuberculosis, trypanosomiasis, onchocerciasis, and malaria. The plan calls for collaboration with other programs and partners in plan development and implementation. MoH staff advised the subcommittee that USAMRU-K participation in this effort would be welcome.

The International Livestock Research Institute possesses an extensive laboratory and is actively engaged in the development of a GIS for Kenya and the African continent. It already uses remote sensing to model epidemics and the distribution of a variety of livestock diseases, a number of which, like Rift Valley fever, trypanosomiasis, and babesiosis, also affect human populations. Many of the data for this work originate from a receiver operated by the Meteorological Department in Nairobi (part of Kenya's Ministry of Natural Resources). This dish receives 1-kilometer-resolution surface temperature and vegetation data from a U.S. National Oceanic and Atmospheric Administration satellite. A team from the National Aeronautics and Space Administration's Goddard Space Center and USAMRU-K recently replaced the receiver.

AMREF, with which USAMRU-K has begun to collaborate, supports a network of more than 120 well-established health care sites in three East African countries and has in place good communication and specimen transport systems. A visit to AMREF headquarters in Nairobi revealed a laboratory of limited capacity with a focus on a medical care-emergency response mission. One of the objectives of AMREF is to support the establishment of a national laboratory program in Kenya. AMREF was established in 1957 with a mission to improve the health of disadvantaged people in Africa. AMREF programs address sexual health, child health, environmental health, health care policy and reform, and clinical services and responses. AMREF is perhaps best known for the latter activity, which is known popularly as "The Flying Doctors." Collaborations with AMREF as part of GEIS include work at Entasopia (dysentery studies) and work in the shantytown of Kibera (urban malaria studies).

USAMRU-K reports that it is beginning to work with MSF. Collaborations with MSF involve surveillance for enteric pathogens and antibiotic resistance at MSF clinic sites in Nairobi slums.

USAMRU-K has informal ties to the CDC. Areas of collaboration include mutual support for the KEMRI Center for Virus Research (a WHO collaborating center), for which USAMRU-K supplies technicians who support the head of the center. The head of the center is in turn supported by the CDC. USAMRU-K also works with the CDC in support of the development of the LIFE Initiative, an AIDS education and prevention program.

USAMRU-K also reports collaborations with the Oxford-Wellcome group on dengue surveillance at Kilifi, environmental change and highland malaria at Kericho, and the molecular pathology of severe pediatric malaria. USAMRU-K also shares HIV-related information with USAID, although they are not active partners. Work with the WHO has focused primarily on support of surveillance for fevers of unknown origin by use of the WHO Yellow Fever Network (a network of sites that was active during the yellow fever epidemic of 1992–1993 in Kenya but that subsequently became inactive and that is now being redeveloped), support for the KEMRI Center for Virus Research, and support for studies of hantavirus and rickettsia. USAMRU-K is not participating directly in a WHO pilot project to develop an integrated disease surveillance network in Kenya. Notably, USAMRU-K is not involved in managing the viral respiratory surveillance and acute febrile illness surveillance projects being conducted by the GEIS Central Hub in Uganda.

## Conclusions

USAMRU-K faces many challenges in a country that is lacking in basic public health and communications infrastructures and that is rife with political difficulties. Nonetheless, its unique geographical location places it in a strategic position to monitor infectious diseases and to achieve GEIS goals. By strengthening and expanding existing partnerships and actively soliciting new partners and collaborators, many of which already support programs that share GEIS's mission, the current USAMRU-K structure can be leveraged to overcome existing hurdles.

Operations in Kenya are very dependent on partnerships, given the relative scarcity of scientific resources. USAMRU-K has a wide variety of existing and potential partners that can assist in accomplishing both research and surveillance objectives. The relationship between USAMRU-K and KEMRI is perhaps the best established. Integration of activities has facilitated collaboration with Kenyan and other visiting scientists. The research centers within KEMRI with which USAMRU-K works offer additional opportunities for collaboration and partnerships that can be used to achieve GEIS goals. The recent transfer of KEMRI to the MoH bodes well for the realization of both the research and the surveillance missions of USAMRU-K. USAMRU-K's location within KEMRI is of benefit to USAMRU-K and offers the possibility for a variety of surveillance activities in support of GEIS goals. Indeed, some of this leveraging has already begun, particularly through work with the Center for Virus Research and the Center for Microbiology Research.

Additional activities can be undertaken to help develop the surveillance infrastructure within Kenya. Of importance to the establishment of a Kenyan public health surveillance system is the direction of more effort to promote the relationship with the MoH. Integral to the provision of surveillance system support is a close working relationship with the central public health agency within the country. The director of the MoH's Communicable Disease Division understands the deficiencies of the current disease reporting system and is eager to work to overcome the lack of infrastructure and to move forward to create an active surveillance system that has the potential to respond to disease epidemics. The epidemiological expertise possessed by the head of the Communicable Disease Control Center would serve GEIS efforts well, and a partnership seems to be worth pursuing. Additionally, providing the MoH with assistance in the development of an epidemic management plan is an activity germane to GEIS and of great potential benefit to Kenya and other in-country partners.

Many of the partnerships that are in place could be expanded. The GIS in development at the International Livestock Research Institute offers exciting potential for the mapping of emerging diseases, such as Rift Valley fever, in Kenya and the surrounding region. MSF and AMREF offer a network of health care facilities throughout the country and throughout Eastern Africa that could be used as a base where active surveillance of priority public health diseases for the country could be initiated or expanded. To the extent that the subcommittee was able to assess its structure, AMREF does not appear to have the capacity or the programmatic interest to conduct basic surveillance activities. AMREF is, however, anxious to obtain support for its ongoing efforts to establish basic diagnostic capabilities within the local clinics that it administers. The laboratory needs of AMREF and the surveillance needs of USAMRU-K may be able to be reconciled to achieve outcomes of benefit to both. The MSF focus on partnership and capacity building corresponds well with GEIS goals. To the extent that these heavily burdened agencies can reliably support USAMRU-K GEIS surveillance efforts, partnerships with both AMREF and MSF would seem to offer valuable opportunities worth actively pursuing.

Insofar as the subcommittee was able to assess the association, it appears that the potential exists for stronger collaboration between USAMRU-K and the CDC for the purposes of emerging infectious disease surveillance. In Kenya, the CDC, like USAMRU-K, has traditionally been oriented to the performance of research rather than the performance of surveillance. However, the CDC is in the process of expanding its staff base in Kenya, and there is a move toward increased surveillance for emerging infectious diseases internationally (Dowell, 2001; Dowell et al., 2001). As such, the sharing of resources and expertise would seem to be in the interests of both partners.

Although the subcommittee was not able to meet with representatives of USAID, the WHO, the Oxford-Wellcome group, or MSF to fully explore existing partnerships and to discuss opportunities for and constraints affecting expanded collaboration, it would appear that each of these organizations, whose missions focus on improving and enhancing public health and infectious disease surveillance throughout the world, represents a potentially valuable collaborator.

As the committee site visit occurred during the early stages of the Ebola virus epidemic in the Gulu District of Uganda, it was particularly evident that close collaborations with and support of the WHO Collaborating Center for Arbovirus and Viral Hemorrhagic Fever Reference and Research and its associated Yellow Fever Surveillance Network are important to USAMRU-K, to Kenya, and throughout the region. Such partnerships present USAMRU-K with an opportunity to strengthen in-country and regional laboratory-based surveillance for viral hemorrhagic fevers and responses to epidemics of viral hemorrhagic fevers. Direct involvement in the WHO integrated disease surveillance project seems to offer the potential to advance GEIS surveillance objectives.

The subcommittee notes, with alarm, the fragmentation of GEIS activities within the region, as evidenced by a lack of coordination and communication between the GEIS Central Hub and USAMRU-K regarding surveillance projects for viral respiratory diseases and acute febrile illnesses in Uganda and Kenya. Such a fragmented approach detracts from the development and presentation of a cohesive GEIS and is damaging to GEIS interests in the long term.

## RECOMMENDATIONS

• GEIS activities at USAMRU-K are of critical importance to the program as a whole. The committee encourages the DoD to plan for GEIS activities at USAMRU-K on a long-term basis. USAMRU-K provides an important resource for both research and surveillance missions. Demand for, and support of, both missions should be balanced so that neither one is jeopardized.

**Recommendation: DoD commitment to GEIS at USAMRU-K should be long term.**

• Current GEIS surveillance activities also work to accomplish outcomes deemed important by the MoH.

**Recommendation: Current GEIS surveillance projects and activities should be continued as they represent activities in support of the GEIS mission.**

• The subcommittee recognizes that the GEIS pillar disease areas are important ones and that defining these targets helps to provide some standardization of GEIS activities across sites, but the pillar structure should be flexible enough to permit local infectious diseases that are of global concern to be addressed as high priorities through GEIS. This serves to take full advantage of the epidemiological setting of the facility, builds national health defenses in the host country, and can be of long-term benefit to the health of many populations, including U.S. military personnel and civilians.

**Recommendation: Consideration should be given to refining the focus of GEIS at USAMRU-K to better enable diseases outside of the pillar areas to be addressed.**

• Consideration needs to be given to expanding existing USAMRU-

K GEIS activities within sub-Saharan Africa, as applicable and as resources permit.

**Recommendation: Expansion of the reach of GEIS activities should be considered.**

• Reagents for the diagnosis of Ebola, Marburg, Crimean-Congo, and Lassa viral hemorrhagic fevers (and other infectious disease entities, as applicable) need to be made consistently and swiftly available to the KEMRI Center for Virus Research to support USAMRU-K surveillance for and response to regionally important pathogens. USAMRU-K relies upon KEMRI for its virology diagnostic capabilities. Without reagents, neither KEMRI nor USAMRU-K will be able to fully support responses to epidemics. Such resources are crucial to the work of GEIS at USAMRU-K and, more generally, to public health surveillance and emerging infectious disease response capacities in Kenya.

**Recommendation: USAMRU-K and the GEIS Central Hub should facilitate the acquisition of reagents for the diagnosis of Ebola, Marburg, Crimean-Congo, and Lassa hemorrhagic fevers (and other infectious disease entities, as applicable) to the extent possible.**

• In addition to reagents, USAMRU-K should have available means of safely, effectively, and rapidly diagnosing regionally important pathogens if it is to fulfill the goals of GEIS. This can be accomplished by improving USAMRU-K laboratory facilities and by forging closer ties with other DoD and non-DoD laboratories.

**Recommendation: Additional GEIS investment in improving USAMRU-K's laboratory capacity is needed and should be pursued within program limits.**

• Effort needs to be made to correct staffing deficiencies and to return USAMRU-K to its authorized contingent of professionals.

**Recommendation: USAMRU-K should have a full-time GEIS program manager on site. The designated GEIS program manager should have training and expertise in applied epidemiology and public health.**

**Recommendation: The assignment of a CDC epidemiologist to USAMRU-K, the assignment of a military public health physician with epidemiological experience, or the assignment of a civilian medical epidemiologist with public health experience should be pursued. To fully realize the GEIS surveillance mission, there should to be strong epidemiological input in USAMRU-K GEIS development and management.**

**Recommendation: USAMRU-K should explore the possibility of supplementing its military scientific staff with Kenyan nationals possessing comparable expertise to ensure continuity of projects, to expand expertise, and to foster collaborative relationships and project growth in important areas of public health surveillance.**

**Recommendation: The availability of staff with virological expertise within USAMRU-K would assist in the achievement of GEIS's goals and should be considered.**

• USAMRU-K needs to work more closely with partners such as the Kenyan MoH, the WHO, USAID, the CDC, and others to strengthen the national surveillance and response capacities for emerging infectious diseases. At the district level, this may include training and the provision of equipment and laboratory support. At the national level, this may include provision of equipment, communications support, and active participation in planning to address emerging infectious diseases.

**Recommendation: Collaborative relationships should continue to be forged and fostered to ensure that USAMRU-K is involved as a full partner in infectious disease surveillance and response activities.**

• Training local personnel in laboratory technology and providing an opportunity for DoD personnel and students to receive research training are important ways in which GEIS is and can increasingly be of benefit to Kenya and the DoD. Consolidating and coordinating USAMRU-K's various training activities under the aegis of GEIS may make training activities more efficient, productive, and visible. The epidemiology training program that USAMRU-K has planned is an important step in these regards. Ultimately, however, a more broadly focused training program that takes full advantage of the expertise and opportunities available at USAMRU-K is desirable. GEIS objectives can be advanced by seeking partnerships with the CDC and other collaborators in training activities. All GEIS training programs in the region need to be part of a cohesive effort.

**Recommendation: DoD and Kenyan training needs should be assessed formally, and the development of a structured USAMRU-K-hosted training program should be considered.**

• Reporting of data on disease incidence is an essential component of a functioning surveillance system. This may take the form of monthly or quarterly reporting of data to the MoH for inclusion in the national or WHO regional surveillance bulletin. Routine reporting needs to be complemented by the development of channels that allow more rapid feedback to the MoH in the event that an epidemic or some other important shift in trends related to a disease agent is detected.

**Recommendation: In consultation with the GEIS Central Hub and public health partners, USAMRU-K should develop and implement a system for the dissemination of public health data in a routine and timely manner to ensure public health action.**

• USAMRU-K GEIS projects need to work together instead of in isolation. All projects in Kenya and the region should operate in coordination with USAMRU-K GEIS activities. Linked projects make relatively efficient use of limited resources and will enhance GEIS visibility.

**Recommendation: Steps should be taken to link GEIS projects together as part of an integrated USAMRU-K GEIS effort.**

• Enhancement of communications infrastructure is an important need that GEIS can help meet. Support for enhancement of communications resources needs to be continued, and a comprehensive plan for improving internal and external networking should be developed.

**Recommendation: Expansion and refined application of communications technologies should be pursued by USAMRU-K with GEIS support.**

• Effort needs be directed to examine GIS output in conjunction with the results of human, vector, and animal studies so that surveillance for malaria and fevers of unknown origin can be enhanced.

**Recommendation: Effort should be directed to enhance the public health application of current GIS work (carried out in collaboration with the International Livestock Research Institute) so that such efforts can better result in information for action.**

• Partnerships benefit from knowledge of the native language by senior staff. Partnerships are of increased importance to USAMRU-K now that its research mission has been formally expanded to include GEIS activities, which necessitate increased interaction with partner agencies. Staff familiarity and comfort with the local language can also improve rates of retention of personnel as well as assist with cultural acclimation.

**Recommendation: Senior staff at USAMRU-K actively involved in GEIS projects should be conversant in the dominant language of the host country or should be encouraged to pursue, with the support of GEIS, language training, and should seek to become conversant to the extent possible.**

## PEOPLE MET AND INTERVIEWED

### *USAMRU-K Staff*

Ronald Rosenberg, commander, USAMRU-K
Raymond Dunton, Malaria Transmission
Jon Davis, clinical laboratory officer, Enteric Pathogens

### *Collaborators and Associates*

Lee Dunster, head, WHO Virus Reference Center, Center for Virological Research, KEMRI
Bernard Ogutu, staff clinician, Center for Clinical Research, KEMRI
Willie Kipkemboi Sang, senior research officer, Center for Microbiology Research, KEMRI
Jane Mbui, research officer, Center for Clinical Research, KEMRI
Joyce Onsongo, director, Division of Communicable Diseases, MoH
Jane Y. Carter, head, Laboratory Programme, African Medical and Research Foundation
Orgenes Lema, chief laboratory technologist, African Medical Research Foundation
Brian D. Perry, veterinary epidemiologist, coordinator, Epidemiology & Disease Control, International Livestock Research Institute
Russ Kruska, GIS analyst, International Livestock Research Institute
Andrew G. Hill, consultant, general surgery; head, Department of Surgery; and director of medical electives, AIC Kijabe Hospital
Kevin DeCock, director, CDC-Kenya
Menique Wasunna, director, Center for Clinical Research, KEMRI

## ITINERARY

### *Monday, October 16*

| | |
|---|---|
| 0930 | Tour of KEMRI |
| 1100 | Briefing (R. Rosenberg) |
| 1200 | Lunch |
| 1400 | Briefing (by L. Dunster in virology and by J. Davis and W. Sang in dysentery) |

### *Tuesday, October 17*

| | |
|---|---|
| 0930 | Ministry of Health: MoH-WHO pilot reportable disease network<br>(J. Onsongo, MoH) |

| | |
|---|---|
| 1200 | Lunch |
| 1300 | AMREF (J. Y. Carter and staff) |
| 1500 | Meet with Koech, director general, KEMRI |

*Wednesday, October 18*

| | |
|---|---|
| 1000 | International Livestock Research Institute (B. D. Perry and R. Kruska, epidemiology and GIS) |
| 1230 | Lunch |
| 1400 | Kijabe Missionary Hospital (L. Dunster and Smith, Yellow Fever Network and rickettsia survey) |

*Thursday, October 19*

| | |
|---|---|
| 0900 | Entasopia dysentery surveillance site (J. Davis, W. Sang, AMREF staff), whole day |

*Friday, October 20*

Depart Kenya

# 7

# GEIS Central Hub and Military Health System Activities

The expanded charge of the Institute of Medicine's (IOM's) Committee to Review the Department of Defense (DoD) Global Emerging Infections Surveillance and Response System states that "the committee will review how well Global Emerging Infections Surveillance and Response System (GEIS) program goals, objectives, and activities are being carried out domestically, namely, within the military health system and the GEIS Central Hub."

The range of GEIS activities addressed within the infrastructure of the military health system (MHS) do not constitute a domestic program per se but are conceptually linked to GEIS as a whole as part of a system of global emerging infectious disease surveillance. As a triservice program, GEIS has taken an approach that pursues gaps in the MHS's capability to identify and address emerging infectious diseases and works to remedy those gaps by building infrastructure, facilitating and supporting response capabilities, providing training and education, and strengthening surveillance capabilities. GEIS resources have been allocated within the MHS to support an array of activities—some new, others already in existence—at many DoD facilities. Together, GEIS laboratory improvement and surveillance activities are intended to "ensure that DoD health care providers have improved access to quality assured, specialized laboratory tests and that those test results are captured for both patient care and public health purposes" (GEIS, 2000b, p. 12).

Within the MHS, many public health surveillance resources are already available. The Army's Center for Health Promotion and Preventive Medicine (CHPPM) maintains a system of databases, the Defense Medical

Surveillance System (DMSS), that provides "up-to-date and historical data on diseases and medical events (e.g., hospitalizations, ambulatory visits, reportable diseases, HIV [human immunodeficiency virus] tests, acute respiratory diseases, and health risk appraisals) and longitudinal data on personnel and deployments" (AMSA, 2001) dating back to 1990 (AMSA, 2001; IOM, 1999). The DoD also maintains a serum repository, linked to the DMSS, that contains more than 20 million specimens (AMSA, 2001). In addition to reporting data to CHPPM,[1] the Navy and the Air Force also maintain distinct surveillance systems, namely, the Naval Disease Reporting System, the Shipboard Non-Tactical ADP (automated data processor) Automated Medical System, and the Air Force Reportable Events Surveillance System (AFRESS). These systems constitute surveillance resources that GEIS seeks to enhance and to make use of in furthering its emerging infectious disease surveillance goals.

To better understand the nature of the domestic and global emerging infections surveillance activities of the DoD, committee members made a site visit to San Diego, California, in January 2001. There the committee visited the Naval Health Research Center (NHRC), as well as the Navy Environmental and Preventive Medicine Unit 5 (NEPMU-5) and the U.S. Naval Hospital, San Diego. Additional information regarding GEIS domestic projects, program management, and collaborative relationships was gathered at a meeting in Washington, D.C., in March 2001. During this meeting, a site visit was made to the U.S. Army Medical Research Institute of Infectious Diseases (USAMRIID). Meeting agendas and lists of people met can be found at the end of this chapter.

To provide the most comprehensive review of a diverse collection of activities possible, this review relies heavily on presented and written material and differs in format from the overseas research laboratory review segments of this report.

## DESCRIPTION OF GEIS CENTRAL HUB AND MHS ACTIVITIES

In the GEIS fiscal year 2000 annual report, GEIS activities are identified as occurring in "three primary settings: the military health system (MHS), the five DoD overseas medical units, and various training, leadership, and capacity building partnerships with regional CINCs [commanders in chief, unified combatant commands] and other governmental and international agencies" (GEIS, 2000b, p. 7).

GEIS operations at the overseas laboratories are considered in detail elsewhere in this report, leaving two areas of GEIS focus to be addressed

---

[1]To date, reporting is incomplete (U.S. Air Force and U.S. Navy comments at presentation to committee, March 2001).

here: activities conducted within the infrastructure of the MHS, and activities conducted in an effort to build partnerships or provide humanitarian assistance (GEIS, 2000b). In addition to these GEIS programmatic activities, the GEIS Central Hub also engages in activities to manage GEIS as a whole.

Core funding for GEIS has been budgeted by using program 8 (P-8) funds—which are operational funds as opposed to research funds. Supplementary funding is also received from unified combatant commands. Through the year 2001, approximately 65 percent of GEIS funds went to support the overseas research laboratories. The remaining funds were divided between the Central Hub, the MHS, and USAMRIID (Kelley, 2001a), as summarized in Tables 7-1 to 7-3.

## GEIS Surveillance-Related Activities

### *General Public Health Laboratory Improvement and Laboratory-Based Surveillance*

**Directory of Laboratory Services and Virtual Public Health Laboratory** In September 1999, GEIS and the Armed Forces Institute of Pathology (AFIP) sponsored a Military Public Health Laboratory Symposium and Workshop, the proceedings of which were published in a supplement to the journal *Military Medicine* (July 2000). The symposium was attended by representatives of academia and members of the public and private sectors. In the course of this symposium, a workshop group convened and considered, as two distinct concepts, the needs and requirements for the development of a DoD Directory of Public Health Laboratory Services and a Virtual Public Health Laboratory (VPHL), respectively (Bolton and Gaydos, 2000).

The DoD Directory of Public Health Laboratory Services was envisioned as a means of making a directory of public health laboratory services for infectious agents available to DoD medical facilities, a resource that the DoD lacks (Bolton and Gaydos, 2000; Gaydos, 2001b). The workshop group contended that clinical, research, environmental, occupational, and veterinary laboratory capacities are not well known to those working outside of each laboratory (Bolton and Gaydos, 2000). As a result, the workshop group states, time can be lost and excessive costs can be incurred when physicians and laboratory personnel make uninformed decisions about where to send specimens for testing (Bolton and Gaydos, 2000; Gaydos, 2001a). Identification of a testing site can be particularly difficult for rare or emerging infectious diseases, as frequently only one laboratory is capable of performing tests (Ascher, 2000). The directory concept also embraces the idea of capturing test results (through the Composite Health Care System [CHCS]) for epidemiological study.

**TABLE 7-1** GEIS Surveillance-Related Activities

| Element | Project or Activity |
|---|---|
| General public health laboratory improvement and laboratory-based surveillance | Virtual Public Health Laboratory |
| | Enhancement of laboratory diagnostic capacity |
| | CHCS implementation |
| Respiratory disease surveillance and capacity building | For example, adenovirus, influenza viruses A and B, *Streptococcus pyogenes*, invasive *Streptococcus pneumoniae* |
| | For example, influenza virus (DoD Laboratory-Based Influenza Surveillance Program) |
| Mortality surveillance | Triservice mortality surveillance |
| Surveillance for and response to sexually transmitted diseases and antibiotic resistance | Gonococcal Isolate Surveillance Project |
| | Antimicrobial resistance surveillance pilot project |
| | Development of a geographic information system for surveillance of sexually transmitted and other diseases |
| Health indicator surveillance | ESSENCE (syndromic surveillance for emerging infectious diseases and bioterrorism events in National Capital Area) |
| | Syndromic surveillance for shipboard deployed forces |

| Lead Agents and Primary Collaborators | GEIS Funding, FY 2000 | Budgeted GEIS Funding, FY 2001[a] | Project Status |
|---|---|---|---|
| AFIP | $60,000 | $320,000[b] | Prototype |
| USAMRIID | $125,000[c] | $135,000[c] | Ongoing |
| Tricare Management Activity | $15,000 | $55,000 | CHCS II in development |
| NHRC | $650,000 | $705,000 | Funded projects under way |
| AFIERA | $508,000 | $590,000 | Ongoing |
| AFIP CHPPM | $100,000 | $105,000[b] | Additional component in development |
| Central Hub in collaboration with CDC, WHO, and domestic and overseas military sites | | $20,000 | Beginning at sentinel site in Hawaii, expansion planned |
| Central Hub in collaboration with Army and Air Force medical centers; CRDA between GEIS, WRAIR, and MRL Pharmaceuticals, Inc. | $64,000 | $60,000 | Beginning at sentinel site in Hawaii, expansion planned |
| Collaboration with USAMRIID and Madigan | $100,000 | $25,000 | One-year pilot beginning in FY 2001; if successful, continued indefinitely |
| Central Hub, CHPPM | $35,000 | $25,000 | Ongoing |
| NEHC | $104,000 | $60,000 | Ongoing |

**TABLE 7-1** Continued

| Element | Project or Activity |
|---|---|
| Malaria and other public health threats in Republic of Korea | Korea malaria/febrile illness surveillance |
| Other Central Hub-managed GEIS projects | Remote sensing |
| | Antimalarial drug surveillance |
| | Surveillance for viral respiratory pathogens and causes of severe acute febrile illnesses in Uganda |
| | Miscellaneous Outbreaks/requested activities (e.g., surveillance for West Nile virus) |

NOTE: FY, fiscal year; CHCS (II), Composite Health Care System (II); AFIP, Armed Forces Institute of Pathology; USAMRIID, U.S. Army Medical Research Institute of Infectious Diseases; NHRC, Naval Health Research Center; AFIERA, Air Force Institute for Environmental Safety and Occupational Health Risk Analysis; ESSENCE, Electronic Surveillance System for the Early Notification of Community-Based Epidemics; CHPPM, Center for Health Promotion and Preventive Medicine, U.S. Army; CDC, U.S. Centers for Disease Control and Prevention; WHO, World Health Organization; CRDA, cooperative research and development agreement; WRAIR, Walter Reed Army Institute of Research; NEHC, Navy Environmental Health Center; MEDCOM, Medical Command; NASA, National Aeronautics and Space Administration; USAMRU-K, U.S. Army Medical Research Unit, Kenya.

The larger VPHL concept—virtual in the sense that it would involve the strengthening and formalization of links between existing laboratories, within and outside of the DoD, not the creation of new facilities—was considered a means of improving lines of communication and coordination, authority, and responsibility within the DoD laboratory system. The VPHL concept incorporates the directory of laboratory services, but it also calls for the strengthening and formation of interlaboratory agreements. The VPHL concept also includes provisions for the collection and archiving of specimens (Bolton and Gaydos, 2000).

The workshop group from the Military Public Health Laboratory Symposium and Workshop emphatically recommended that a World Wide Web-based DoD Directory of Public Health Laboratory Services be

| Lead Agents and Primary Collaborators | GEIS Funding, FY 2000 | Budgeted GEIS Funding, FY 2001[a] | Project Status |
|---|---|---|---|
| 18th MEDCOM | $100,000 | $75,000 | Ongoing |
| Collaboration with NASA | $10,000 | $40,000 | Under way |
| Collaboration with WRAIR and WHO | 0 | $60,000 | Ongoing |
| Collaboration with AFIERA, WRAIR, WHO, Uganda Viral Research Institute, USAMRU-K, Rakai Project | 0 | $60,000 | Under development |
| Collaborations as needed or directed | $40,000 | $47,600 | Projects conducted as needed |

[a]Preliminary budget estimates as of August 8, 2000. Figures are subject to change throughout the fiscal year and are provided only to give the reader a general sense of the scope and scale of GEIS project activity. These figures should not be interpreted as exact expenditures.

[b]Estimated figures per S. Gubenia, Department of Defense Global Emerging Infections Surveillance and Response System, June 21, 2001.

[c]Direct GEIS funding. Additional GEIS funds are provided indirectly through the laboratories for the processing of specimens and other services.

SOURCES: GEIS, 2000a,b,c; Kelley, 2001b.

developed. The workshop group advised that responsibility for operating, evaluating, and updating the directory should rest with AFIP, in coordination with GEIS. Rather than supporting the separate development of the directory and VPHL concepts, the workshop group viewed the directory as the first step in the realization of VPHL goals. The workshop group also suggested that some of the perceived weaknesses in the laboratory system could be addressed through alternative means, such as pursuit of formal agreements (i.e., with the U.S. Centers for Disease Control and Prevention [CDC]). The recommendations of the workshop group were subsequently endorsed by the Armed Forces Epidemiology Board (AFEB) (AFEB, 2000).

A prototype of the DoD Directory of Public Health Laboratory Ser-

**TABLE 7-2** GEIS Training and Development Activities

| Element | Project or Activity | Agent | GEIS Funding, FY 2000 | Budgeted GEIS Funding, FY 2001[a] | Status |
|---|---|---|---|---|---|
| Training and capacity building | Overseas Medical Research Laboratory Orientation Training Program | Central Hub | $50,000 | $100,000 | Ongoing |
| | Peruvian Laboratory-Based Public Health Surveillance Project[b] | Central Hub, Instituto Nacional de Salud | $105,000 | Unknown | Ongoing |
| | Caribbean Laboratory-Based Public Health Surveillance Project[b] | Central Hub, WRAIR, CAREC | | | Ongoing |
| | U.S. Army Health Facilities Planning Agency Support to the Caribbean Epidemiology Center[b] | Central Hub, HFPA, CAREC | | | Ongoing |
| Systems research, development, and integration (infrastructure development) | GEIS website (GEISWeb) | Central Hub | $75,000 | | Ongoing |

NOTE: FY, fiscal year; WRAIR, Walter Reed Army Institute of Research; CAREC, Caribbean Epidemiology Center; HFPA, Health Facilities Planning Agency.

[a]Preliminary budget estimates as of August 8, 2000. Figures are subject to change throughout the fiscal year and are provided only to give the reader a general sense of the scope and scale of GEIS project activity. These figures should not be interpreted as exact expenditures.

[b]Supported with funds supplied by the Overseas, Humanitarian, Disaster, and Civil Aid (OHDACA) program.

SOURCES: GEIS, 2000a,b,c; Kelley, 2001b.

**TABLE 7-3** GEIS Management Activities

| Element | Project or Activity | Agent | GEIS Funding, FY 2000 | Budgeted GEIS Funding, FY 2001[a] | Status |
|---|---|---|---|---|---|
| Management | Develop, coordinate, and monitor execution of strategic plan | | | | |
| | Review annual proposals for funding and prioritize support | | | | |
| | Coordinate distribution of funds | | | | |
| | Review and publish annual reports from GEIS funded agencies | | | | |
| | Assist with obtaining supplementary resources | | | | |
| | Represent GEIS to higher headquarters and other federal, international, and local agencies | | | | |
| | Facilitate CINC-supported civic assistance projects | | | | |
| | Manage public and professional awareness initiatives | | | | |
| | Foster solutions to emerging infections problems through sponsorship of professional forums | | | | |
| | TOTAL | Central Hub | $715,000 | $715,000 | Ongoing |

NOTE: FY, fiscal year; CINC, commander in chief, unified combatant command.

[a]Preliminary budget estimates as of August 8, 2000. Figures are subject to change throughout the fiscal year and are provided only to give the reader a general sense of the scope and scale of GEIS activity.

SOURCES: GEIS, 2000b,c; Kelley, 2001b.

vices was presented to the IOM committee at its meeting in March 2001. The "first-step" product is to offer a World Wide Web-based listing of participating laboratories, available laboratory tests, charges for tests (if any), points of contact within participating laboratories, specimen submission procedures, and reporting procedures (Kalasinsky, 2001). With planned additions, the directory will move to increasingly encompass the VPHL concept and is to offer regular updates (monthly), realistic turnaround times for tests, toxicology results, patient records, or test results (in a secure, access-limited area), and access to the frozen specimen repository (Kalasinsky, 2001). No plans are in place to make the directory available to non-DoD users.

Ultimately, however, non-DoD laboratories are also envisioned as playing a role in VPHL (Bolton and Gaydos, 2000). Potential partners in what is to evolve to become VPHL include the following (Kelley, 2001a):

- clinical treatment facility laboratories;
- the Walter Reed Army Institute of Research (WRAIR), USAMRIID, and DoD overseas laboratories;
- Brooks Air Force Base (Project Gargle);
- NHRC laboratory;
- CHPPM laboratories;
- TAML [theater area medical laboratories] and other advanced forward laboratories;
- DoD veterinary pathology laboratories;
- AFIP;
- CDC and selected state health department laboratories; and
- academic institutions.

**Enhancement of Laboratory Capacity** USAMRIID serves as a reference center for the isolation and identification of infectious disease agents requiring handling at biosafety level 3 and above. USAMRIID serves as a DoD and World Health Organization (WHO) reference center for the testing of human specimens for unusual infectious disease agents. GEIS supports the USAMRIID infrastructure as a means of maintaining capacity for emerging infectious disease surveillance and response. This support is provided on the basis of the assertion that a broad, operationally oriented DoD reference laboratory for the isolation and identification of unusual etiologic agents and the diagnosis of infectious diseases requiring high levels of containment is in the interest of GEIS (GEIS, 2000b). GEIS at USAMRIID contributes to surveillance capabilities by producing, testing, and stockpiling critical diagnostic reagents to support surveillance and epidemic investigations of global emerging infections. In fiscal year 2000, USAMRIID needed and produced reagents for the detection of infection due to hantavirus, tick-borne encephalitis viruses, dengue virus,

Venezuelan equine encephalomyelitis virus, West Nile virus, St. Louis encephalitis virus, Crimean Congo hemorrhagic fever virus, Marburg virus, anthrax, brucellosis, tularemia, and other infectious diseases and infectious disease agents (GEIS, 2000b). These reagents were widely distributed within the DoD and in some cases to civilian collaborators. USAMRIID also undertook the production of non-cross-reactive diagnostic reagents for West Nile virus as part of the DoD response to a request from the CDC for assistance with surveillance for West Nile virus.

USAMRIID also plays a role in the training of both DoD and civilian personnel in the performance of diagnostic techniques and procedures, as needed (GEIS, 2000b). In addition to the funds directly provided to USAMRIID by GEIS for capacity-building purposes, USAMRIID also receives support from GEIS indirectly through laboratories that seek USAMRIID services for, for instance, entomological studies and confirmation of diagnoses.

**CHCS** GEIS has set aside funds to support the development of capabilities within CHCS II, the successor to CHCS, a clinical information system project that began in the early 1980s. The DoD's CHCS consists of databases maintained at medical treatment facilities worldwide. These databases contain information on the results of laboratory test results and pharmacy data. However, these databases are not linked together as part of a cohesive system. To overcome limitations associated with this disconnect, a linked system, CHCS II, is in development and will be used to support laboratory-based surveillance activities (GEIS, 2000b; IOM, 1999).

At present, DoD laboratories, as opposed to health care providers, are not required to report notifiable infections to DoD authorities, although they are required report the occurrence of such infections to civilian public health authorities (Frommelt, 2000; Brady and Frommelt, 2000; IOM, 1999). However, at the Military Public Health Laboratory Symposium and Workshop held in September 1999, the workshop group recommended that all requests for testing made as part of the DoD Directory of Public Health Laboratory Services be entered into the DoD's laboratory information system, the CHCS (or CHCS II), to create an audit trail for test requests, to make results quickly available to those with system access, and to promote proper archiving of data (Bolton and Gaydos, 2000). GEIS envisions that such a mechanism of rapid laboratory-based reporting through CHCS will also enable the tracking of the incidence of important infections and antibiotic resistance, the goal being the prompt detection of all cases that warrant a public health response (GEIS, 1998).

*Respiratory Disease Surveillance and Capacity Building*

GEIS MHS respiratory disease surveillance efforts are primarily focused within the NHRC in San Diego California, and the Air Force Institute for Environmental Safety and Occupational Health Risk Analysis (AFIERA), centered at Brooks Air Force Base in San Antonio, Texas. NHRC and AFIERA are the Navy and Air Force "hubs" (coordinating units) for GEIS within the MHS, respectively. GEIS, in seeking to build upon and coordinate existing DoD laboratory expertise, has identified facilities that possess particularly robust capabilities in a specified area. GEIS has identified the NHRC as a center of expertise and excellence in the area of respiratory viruses and bacteria and surveillance for acute respiratory diseases in military training centers. AFIERA has been designated a center of expertise and excellence in the areas of influenza and tuberculosis (Gaydos, 1999). In addition to providing funds to support projects, GEIS resources also support laboratory capacity building within these hubs.

**NHRC** The NHRC laboratory is a biosafety level 2 facility that possesses virology-, bacteriology-, and molecular biology-based study components. The NHRC conducts for DoD national surveillance for adenovirus, influenza viruses A and B, *Streptococcus pyogenes*, and invasive *Streptococcus pneumoniae* at U.S. Army, Navy, Marine Corps, Air Force, and Coast Guard sites identified as "high risk." The laboratory's work involves 17 collaborating military commands. Laboratory staff conduct surveillance for the emergence of new pathogenic strains and the development of antibiotic resistance. The laboratory team also follows large cohorts of military personnel in prospective epidemiological studies of respiratory disease and conducts large clinical trials of interventions for the prevention or treatment of respiratory diseases (NHRC, 2001b).

In fiscal year 2000, GEIS funds supported numerous NHRC project activities involving surveillance, evaluation of new diagnostic tools, identification of risk factors for respiratory diseases, and epidemic investigations (GEIS, 2000b). GEIS also provides capacity that the NHRC has been able to leverage to conduct research activities such as clinical trials. Ongoing and recently completed NHRC epidemiological studies of emerging illness among U.S. military personnel (supported to various degrees by GEIS) include the following (GEIS, 2000b; NHRC, 2001a,c; Ryan et al., 2000):

- triservice surveillance for *S. pyogenes* infections among U.S. military personnel;
- triservice surveillance for antibiotic resistance among *S. pneumoniae* isolates infecting U.S. military health care beneficiaries;
- triservice population-based surveillance for viral respiratory pathogens among high-risk military personnel;

- epidemiological study of respiratory diseases among midshipmen at the U.S. Naval Academy;
- double-blind, placebo-controlled clinical trial of azithromycin as prophylaxis against bacterial agents causing acute respiratory disease among military trainees;
- clinical evaluation of a rapid diagnostic test for adenovirus;
- clinical evaluation of two rapid diagnostic tests for influenza virus;
- double-blind, placebo-controlled clinical efficacy trial of pneumococcal vaccine or benzathine penicillin G as prophylaxis against bacterial agents causing febrile acute respiratory disease among ranger trainees;
- double-blind, placebo-controlled trial of the 23-valent pneumococcal vaccine among military trainees at high risk of respiratory disease;
- surveillance for *Bordetella pertussis* among military trainees with respiratory disease;
- an evaluation of screening results for tuberculosis among young adults enlisting in the U.S. Navy;
- evaluation of military recruit populations for respiratory syncytial virus infection;
- clinical evaluation of Zstatflu and Directigen, two rapid diagnostic tests for influenza virus; and
- development and support of unique virology and bacteriology capabilities and studies.

The NHRC has also participated in collaborative epidemic response efforts outside of the military population, upon request (e.g., identification of respiratory disease in Tijuana, Mexico, in collaboration with Mexican and Californian public health authorities) (NHRC, 2000a,c). The NHRC maintains a website that provides detailed information about ongoing and recently completed projects. This site is linked to the GEIS website (GEISWeb). The NHRC also produces a periodic GEIS Respiratory Disease Surveillance Newsletter that provides project information and updates and is publicly accessible on the Internet.

**AFIERA** Within the Air Force hub, AFIERA, GEIS support is focused particularly on influenza (Neville and Canas, 2001). The Air Force is the executive agent for DoD surveillance for influenza (Bailey, 1999) and the Air Force influenza surveillance program has existed for more than 20 years. Presidential Decision Directive NSTC-7 (NSTC, 1996), coupled with GEIS funding, fueled program expansion in 1998. The Air Forces's etiology-based surveillance program, formerly called Project Gargle, is now the Department of Defense Laboratory-Based Influenza Surveillance Program, in which 19 global sentinel sites, 49 nonsentinel sites, and 3 DoD overseas medical research laboratories participate (GEIS, 2000b, 2001e).

AFIERA is an active collaborator in the WHO influenza surveillance laboratory at the CDC and provides input to the U.S. Food and Drug Administration regarding annual influenza vaccine components (Canas et al., 2000). In 1999, AFIERA was able to isolate and subtype a strain of the influenza A virus (H3N2), which was subsequently forwarded to the CDC and became the seed virus for the 2000–2001 and 2001–2002 vaccine component (Gaydos, 2001d). Also of note, AFIERA's work with the Naval Medical Research Center Detachment, Peru, identified the presence of an influenza virus strain (H1N1) in the Americas, and led to its inclusion in the influenza vaccines for both the Northern and Southern Hemispheres during both the 2000–2001 and 2001–2002 flu seasons. AFIERA surveillance also covers people living in proximity to overseas DoD research facilities, as well as military personnel. AFIERA is also working to conduct studies to evaluate the clinical effectiveness of influenza vaccine in military personnel (GEIS, 2000b).

To more effectively disseminate surveillance findings, AFIERA produces influenza activity reports for sentinel and nonsentinel sites, updated biweekly, and has made them available on its website (monthly summary information is available to nongovernment users), which is linked to GEISWeb. GEIS-supported, AFIERA-managed activities also include additional surveillance work (e.g., trainee health surveillance and West Nile virus surveillance), provision of support for epidemic investigations (e.g., acute febrile illness among trainees at Lackland Air Force Base, Texas), support and enhancement of existing programs (e.g., AFRESS and molecular biology capabilities), and special studies (e.g., case-control study of influenza vaccine and chlamydia prevalence study) (GEIS, 2000b; Neville and Canas, 2001).

AFIERA GEIS program accomplishments in fiscal year 2000 include the following (GEIS, 2000b, p. 79):

- implementation of a record validation program for communicable disease reports to ensure records meet the criteria specified for DMSS;
- design of layout for World Wide Web-based interactive reports on reportable events;
- conversion of AFRESS influenza reporting from routine to urgent;
- implementation of weekly influenza activity reports for each sentinel site as well as for nonsentinel sites;
- design of layout for World Wide Web-based interactive reports for influenza surveillance;
- establishment of protocols and data collection mechanisms for influenza vaccine effectiveness study;
- molecular biology-based protocols for extraction of RNA;
- expanded surveillance efforts to include genetic characterization of neuraminidase;
- retrieval of command support for chlamydia prevelance study; and

- evaluation of adenovirus outbreak at Lackland Air Force Base.

*Mortality Surveillance*

In 1997, recognizing the lack of a comprehensive DoD system for mortality surveillance, the Armed Forces Epidemiology Board formally recommended the institution of mortality surveillance within the DoD. In response, the Uniformed Services University of the Health Sciences (USUHS) and the AFIP, funded by GEIS, developed a registry that will permit more timely capture of data in integrated databases, allowing long-term analysis (through the triservice database, DMSS). The registry as presently constructed, however, does not include an emerging infectious disease alert component, a feature that is important to GEIS. GEIS is working with AFIP to add an emerging infectious disease alert component to the DoD Epidemiology and Mortality Surveillance System and associated Mortality Registry (Gardner et al., 2000).

The alert component will serve to rapidly identify deaths possibly attributable to emerging infectious disease agents, based on uniform criteria for the identification of suspicious cases of illness. The identification of a death suspected of being caused by an emerging infectious disease will trigger a rapid investigation, beginning with telephone contact with the attending physician to determine whether a specific investigation of the diagnosis is required and to identify specimens that might need to be forwarded for sophisticated laboratory examination at both DoD and non-DoD laboratories. The Armed Forces Medical Examiner is to be charged with responding to "red flags" raised by this system (Gaydos, 2001c). Although GEIS is providing funding and guidance for the development of the emerging infectious disease alert component, ultimately the registry will be maintained by the AFIP and CHPPM.

*Surveillance for and Response to STDs and Antibiotic Resistance*

**GIS Development and STD Surveillance** On the basis of the success at Ft. Bragg, North Carolina, in which geographic information systems (GISs) were used to track sexually transmitted diseases (STDs) and gastrointestinal illnesses, GEIS is providing funding for implementation of a similar effort at Ft. Lewis, Washington (GEIS, 2000b; Gunzenhauser, 2000). Although STDs are the diseases of focus, the larger purposes of this work are (1) to develop a GIS-based surveillance system that can be used as an epidemic investigation tool (GEIS, 2000b) and (2) to assess the validity of immediately reported outpatient data (like the data used in the Electronic Surveillance System for the Early Notification of Community-Based Epidemics [ESSENCE], a project for syndromic surveillance for emerging infectious diseases and bioterrorism events in the National Capital Area) by comparing it with CHCS laboratory data (Gunzenhauser, 2000). Evaluating the feasibility and value of sharing data with local civilian health officials is also a planned part of this pilot project. The project is being coordinated with the GEIS ESSENCE project (Gunzenhauser, 2000).

**GISP** GEIS is working with the CDC to add additional sites to the CDC Gonococcal Isolate Surveillance Project (GISP), a CDC-sponsored active surveillance program designed to track changes and reveal trends in antibiotic resistance in *Neisseria gonorrhoeae*. Within the MHS, surveillance will focus on the DoD beneficiary population at both domestic and non-U.S. locations. The overseas medical laboratory component of this work calls for collaboration with the WHO and other countries for surveillance in foreign national populations (GEIS, 2000b). The first DoD site chosen for addition to the network was Tripler Army Medical Center in Hawaii due to a recent increase in the incidence of drug-resistant gonococcal organisms in Hawaii.

**Antibiotic Resistance Surveillance** To advance antibiotic resistance surveillance activities within the DoD, GEIS has also established a cooperative research and development agreement with MRL, Inc., to test automated approaches for standardized, real-time antibiotic resistance surveillance at several DoD health care facilities (GEIS, 2000b). Participating DoD facilities enroll as sentinel sites with MRL. Resistance data are then submitted to MRL and subjected to an "extensive quality assessment process." Participating sites can query the MRL database, The Surveillance Network Database (GEIS, 2001g), via a secure connection to the World Wide Web for information pertinent to their site and to compare statistics for the site with regional and national data. Data can be shared between sites and with the Central Hub. One DoD site (Wilford Hall Air Force Medical Center) has already begun participating in this arrangement. Two other sites (Tripler Army Medical Center and Keesler Air Force Medical Center) are in the process of developing agreements (GEIS, 2000b).

### *Health Indicator Surveillance*

**ESSENCE** The Electronic Surveillance System for the Early Notification of Community-Based Epidemics (ESSENCE) has been a focus of GEIS health indicator surveillance funding. ESSENCE was developed by the GEIS Central Hub in collaboration with CHPPM and numerous other agencies and academic institutions. This program is intended to detect emerging infectious disease epidemics, including bioterrorist events, for the purposes of instigating a timely response, promoting rapid epidemiology-based targeting of limited response assets (e.g., personnel and drugs), and equipping leaders in civil government to communicate risk on the basis of estimates of levels of exposure to reduce the spread of panic and unrest (GEIS, 2001d; Pavlin, 2000, 2001a).

To date, efforts have focused largely on the National Capital Area, which has more than 100 DoD primary health care clinics. As part of the project, ESSENCE receives ambulatory care data on a daily basis from the Ambulatory Data System currently in place at all continental U.S. military treatment facilities (data are collected by the Tricare Management Agency). Data are aggregated into syndrome groups on the basis of the codes in the International Classification of Diseases, 9th edition. These syndromic clusters are monitored for changes in incidence or clustering of cases of illness that could signal an emerging infectious disease event. A geographic information component of the system developed by CHPPM is used to plot cases for graphic assessment. Collaborative input has been sought from the Washington Metropolitan Council of Government's Subcommitee on Public Health and local universities (GEIS, 2000b). ESSENCE is still in development. To date, data feeds from reporting locations have been established, basic trend analyses with historical data have been produced, the basic GIS mapping component has been developed, and partnerships for the sharing of data have been cultivated (Pavlin, 2001a). GEIS's work on the development of this and other surveillance systems spawned the Conference and Workshop on Syndromic and Other Surveillance Methods for Emerging Infections held in May 2001 (GEIS, 2000b).

**NEHC** The Navy Environmental Health Center (NEHC) receives funding from GEIS to improve syndromic and other surveillance capabilities for its shipboard deployed forces and special forces personnel. U.S. Navy and U.S. Marine Corps forces are continuously deployed to remote regions throughout the world and thus are at increased risk of encountering emerging infectious diseases. In particular, the focus of GEIS at NEHC has been on the merging of two existing surveillance systems, the Naval Disease Reporting System and the Shipboard Non-Tactical ADP Automated Medical System. Integration of the two systems is to result in one system that is administered by the Space and Information Warfare Center but through which data are channeled to NEHC epidemiologists for analysis and response. Systems integration is intended to provide direct and smooth acquisition of shipboard surveillance data (a function that is available to other medical settings within the Navy and the Marine Corps) and to make data more useful for syndromic surveillance purposes. An effort has also been directed to the development of sentinel (nonshipboard) surveillance sites in areas where personnel are deployed (e.g., a training site in Ecuador), and data sharing and epidemiological support relationships with the host country and Naval Medical Research Center Detachment, Peru (NMRCD) are being cultivated (Morrow, 2000;

Murphy, 2001). Ultimately, plans are to deploy the combined Naval Disease Reporting System/Shipboard Non-Tactical ADP Automated Medical System at sentinel sites as well.

GEIS also sponsors a separate surveillance activity, conducted by Navy Environmental and Preventive Medicine Units 2 (NEPMU-2) and 5 (NEPMU-5) (subordinate commands of NEHC) in collaboration with Naval Medical Research Unit 2 (NAMRU-2), for viral gastroenteritis surveillance aboard deployed Navy vessels. This work focuses on the detection and identification of shipboard epidemics and the development of methods, tools, and protocols for case identification and response (Thornton, 2001), predominantly for the Norwalk and Norwalk-like viral agents. NEPMU-5 is also seeking to become a DoD reference laboratory for enteric pathogens. NEPMU-5 has also indicated an interest in operating as the DoD laboratory hub or center of excellence for enteric pathogens (Thornton, 2000).

### *Malaria and Other Public Health Threats in Republic of Korea*

GEIS has provided partial support for 18th Medical Command (MEDCOM) projects in the Republic of Korea. GEIS funding has been used to improve field, nonhuman surveillance capabilities in the 18th MEDCOM. The recent reemergence of vivax malaria in South Korea and ongoing morbidity in both South Korean and U.S. troops provides particular motivation for this support. Adult and larval mosquitoes are trapped, processed, and analyzed (by enzyme-linked immunosorbent assay) with some support from the Armed Forces Research Institute of Medical Sciences (AFRIMS), to identify areas of transmission and relative risks. Surveillance of mosquitoes for Japanese encephalitis virus and surveillance of rodents for rodent-borne diseases (diseases caused by Hantaan and Seoul viruses, scrub typhus, murine typhus, and leptospirosis) are also conducted in collaboration with USAMRIID and Korea University. Work is also under way to identify high-risk breeding sites for mosquitoes, to assess the knowledge of soldiers serving in the area regarding personal protective measures, and to explore the relationship between compliance with prophylaxis and occurrence of possible drug resistance (Klein and Lee, 2001). Health data supplied by CHPPM, the Korean National Institutes of Health, and the Republic of Korea Military are also being used to identify trends in the prevalence of vivax malaria in U.S. forces, Republic of Korea forces, and civilians in surrounding communities (Klein and Lee, 2001).

Potential tick-borne diseases are also being investigated in U.S. military personnel. Additional tick surveillance will provide an analysis of potential human pathogens associated with sites where U.S. forces train in Korea. This work is conducted in collaboration with the Korean National Institutes of Health and Chanbuk University, Korea.

*Other Central Hub-Managed Projects*

**Remote Sensing (Collaborations with NASA)** GEIS collaborates with the National Aeronautics and Space Administration (NASA) on the use of satellite-based remote sensing to predict epidemic infectious diseases. Although the field is still in its infancy, results to date have been quite encouraging. Most of the collaboration is with the Goddard Space Flight Center, but GEIS also collaborates with several other agencies. The objectives of the program are to identify links between the environment and emerging diseases, develop methods to detect linked environmental events by remote sensing, conduct surveillance, predict emerging infectious diseases by use of remote sensing, and publish maps of areas of risk on the World Wide Web for use by the WHO and other agencies. Remote sensing is particularly suited to this type of problem because it may be the only technology capable of realistically conducting surveillance continually over time and over large geographical areas. The technique has been used to identify close coupling between ecology (remotely sensed vegetation index), interannual climate variability such as that brought about by the El Niño-Southern Oscillation, and epidemics of Rift Valley fever in East Africa. The mechanism is thought to be due to an effect of rainfall on flooding and the hatching and emergence of the mosquito vectors of Rift Valley fever. The remote-sensing profiles used to draw these associations have been used to create and publish, on a monthly basis, maps of areas in continental Africa, Madagascar, and the Arabian Peninsula at risk for Rift Valley fever. A similar method is being developed to conduct surveillance for conditions favorable to the occurrence of epidemics, including epidemics of Ebola and Marburg viruses, in Africa. Preliminary data suggest that a similar approach may be used to develop maps of areas in Southeast Asia at risk for dengue hemorrhagic fever (Linthicum, 2001).

**WRAIR WHO Center for Antimalarial Drug Surveillance** For more than 30 years, Military Infectious Disease Research Program (MIDRP)-supported malaria research projects have been under way. These projects are based at WRAIR and capitalize on the opportunities afforded by the overseas research laboratories. These projects have emphasized and contributed greatly to antimalarial drug discovery and development. GEIS seeks to add to the existing capacity by enhancing mechanisms for the timely and systematic exchange of laboratory specimens between the overseas laboratories and public health partners (Milhous et al., 2000). To accomplish this, GEIS is partnering with the Multilateral Initiative for Malaria (MIM).[2]

In 1999, after a WHO workshop, "Markers of Antimalarial Drug Resistance: Practical, Clinical, and Epidemiological Applications," a National Institute of Allergy and Infectious Diseases grant was issued to sponsor, in support of MIM, the development of the Malaria Research and Reference Reagent Repository, a repository designed to improve access to reagents for the evaluation of parasites, vectors, and humans and to promote the standardization of assays with well-characterized and renewable reagents (Milhous et al., 2000; MIMCom, 2001). WRAIR's Division of Experimental Therapeutics has been identified as the focal point for GEIS surveillance and detection of drug-resistant malaria (Milhous et al., 2000). As a partner in MIM, GEIS contributes funds in support of research projects at WRAIR and at the overseas laboratories (Milhous et al., 2000).

**Surveillance for Viral Respiratory Pathogens and Causes of Severe Acute Febrile Illness in Uganda** GEIS surveillance for viral respiratory pathogens and for severe acute febrile illnesses is planned in Uganda. As part of the viral respiratory pathogen surveillance study, individuals who present at the Rakai Project Clinic (Rakai District, Uganda) with fever will be sampled for influenza A and B viruses; parainfluenza virus types 1, 2, and 3; adenovirus; enterovirus; and herpes virus. Samples will be sent to Brooks Air Force Base for testing. This project is intended to improve influenza surveillance efforts in sub-Saharan Africa, an area largely undercovered in terms of international surveillance for influenza. Surveillance for severe acute febrile illnesses is to be conducted in Kalisizo Hospital (Rakai District, Uganda). Laboratory testing is to involve the efforts of an on-site project technician, U.S. Army Medical Research Unit, Kenya (USAMRU-K), and the WHO. Project reports are to be sent to the GEIS Central Hub and relevant collaborators. Though this work has been in development for some time, neither project has been implemented as both projects have yet to receive approval from appropriate governmental authorities (Pavlin, 2001b).

---

[2]MIM is a partnership of organizations and individuals that are concerned about malaria, particularly malaria in Africa. The National Institutes of Health Fogarty International Center serves as the secretariat of the alliance, although the Wellcome Trust has served in this capacity in the past. MIM is funded primarily by the National Institute of Allergy and Infectious Diseases, the WHO Special Program for Research and Training in Tropical Diseases (which administers MIM scientific projects), the World Bank, the Rockefeller Foundation, and the Roll Back Malaria campaign; but it includes the partnership of many research institutes, research funding agencies, foundations, and control agencies, as well as the United Nations (through several WHO programs) (MIMCom, 2001).

**Miscellaneous Outbreaks and Projects** The GEIS Central Hub maintains contingency funds to support emerging infectious disease response efforts, as needed, and to conduct surveillance projects that are time sensitive (i.e., that cannot wait for the next funding cycle).

For instance, in fiscal year 2000 one contingency activity included surveillance for West Nile virus. At the request of the CDC, the GEIS Central Hub coordinated the reporting of DoD human, bird, and mosquito surveillance data and represented the DoD in weekly conference calls with the CDC and state West Nile virus coordinators (GEIS, 2000b). As part of DoD activities for surveillance for West Nile virus, extensive mosquito surveillance was conducted by CHPPM along the East Coast, information on suspected human cases (none were confirmed) was supplied by Walter Reed Army Medical Center, the North Atlantic Veterinary Command coordinated the testing of birds (four birds were found to be positive for West Nile virus), and the Air Force reported extensive data obtained by the trapping of mosquitoes. Further DoD participation in the West Nile virus surveillance effort is contingent on national plans (GEIS, 2000b).

Also, through participation in military medical conferences, AFEB and IOM meetings, meetings of the Joint Preventive Medicine Policy Group and other staff meetings, and review of documents, GEIS attempts to identify emerging infectious disease problem areas, document these problems, develop an awareness regarding the problems, and develop and recommend solutions and foster the implementation and evaluation of interventions. Examples of this are the studies, publications, and presentations on acute respiratory diseases in the military that have been used to (1) inform the DoD, the military leadership, AFEB, and IOM; (2) to educate health care providers; and (3) to assist the U.S. Army Medical Research Acquisition Activity and the U.S. Army Medical Research and Materiel Command to develop requests for proposals for adenovirus vaccine development and means for evaluating the proposals (Gaydos, 2001e). Similarly, studies, publications, and presentations on STDs in the military have been used to inform the DoD, the military leadership, and AFEB and to educate health care providers (GEIS, 2000b; Gaydos, 2001e). GEIS has facilitated and fostered the development of an AFEB recommendation on screening for chlamydial infection, reports from the DoD STD Prevention Committee to the DoD medical and nonmedical leadership, the exchange of data and information on STDs among the services, and initiatives to improve STD programs for the Air Force and Coast Guard (Gaydos, 2001e).

## GEIS Training and Development Activities

*Training and Capacity Building*

**Overseas Medical Research Laboratory Orientation Training Program** The Overseas Medical Research Laboratory Orientation Training Program has as its objectives "to expand the cadre of DoD personnel with an interest in pursuing a career in tropical public health surveillance and research with a particular focus on emerging infections" (Writer, 2001b). Trainees are selected from among those who are already on active duty with the DoD, who are interested in international infectious disease work, and who are willing to consider assignment at one of the overseas research laboratories. Interested individuals are encouraged to identify the location where they would like to work, the subject of their project, and the potential time that they are available. Selected individuals work with laboratory staff on research or public health projects that are being conducted by the laboratory (GEIS, 2000b). The first team was selected in late 1999, and by the end of fiscal year 2000 a total of 16 students had been funded for an average length of rotation of 39 days. Continued training cycles are planned in 2001 (Writer, 2001b).

**Peruvian Laboratory-Based Public Health Surveillance Project** Using humanitarian assistance funds from the U.S. Southern Command (SOUTHCOM), the GEIS Central Hub has provided computers (5 in the year 2000 and 15 to date, with additional donations planned) and software to the Peruvian Instituto Nacional de Salud (INS; Peruvian National Institutes of Health) to facilitate transmission of data between local, regional, and national facilities. The Central Hub has also provided training to INS personnel in the use of CDC's Public Health Laboratory Information System. The goals of this effort are to assist the Peruvian national health system in developing a laboratory-based surveillance system and, ultimately, a locally sustainable electronic disease and syndromic surveillance system in Peru. Humanitarian assistance funds for this project are being contributed by SOUTHCOM (GEIS, 2000b; Writer, 2001a).

**Caribbean Laboratory-Based Public Health Surveillance Project and U.S. Army Health Facilities Planning Agency Support to the Caribbean Epidemiology Center** In 1996, WRAIR staff, dispatched to the Caribbean region at the request of the Atlantic Command, determined that the existing public health surveillance capacity was insufficient (Writer, 2001b). After the introduction of GEIS, the Caribbean Laboratory-Based Public Health Surveillance Project was developed to assist the Caribbean Epidemiology Center (CAREC; a center of the Pan American Health Organization's Division of Disease Prevention and Control) in assembling a computerized network to support disease surveillance and communication among CAREC's 21 member nations (GEIS, 2000b, 2001b). GEIS, with SOUTHCOM and Atlantic Command funding, has provided computers, software, and training in basic computer use and surveillance systems (the CDC's Public Health Laboratory Information System) in support of this effort to assemble an Internet-based regional computerized surveillance network. GEIS Central Hub staff have made repeated trips to the region to provide equipment and training. To date, 145 computers have been donated. In addition, as many as 250 public health workers from CAREC member countries have received basic instruction in computer use and surveillance systems and about 200 workers have received more advanced training (GEIS, 2000b). Currently, 24 sites in 10 countries are participating in the network, and the network continues to grow as individuals trained as a part of this project are now able to train others with minimal input from CAREC staff.

Also, at the request of the U.S. ambassador in Trinidad and Tobago, SOUTHCOM, GEIS, WRAIR, the U.S. Army Health Facilities Planning Agency, and CAREC worked together to assess current CAREC laboratory and administrative space to document structural and safety planning needs and to begin the design of a new 64,000-square-foot facility. The initial survey product has led the government of Trinidad and Tobago to commit $400,000 (U.S.) to begin detailed design (GEIS, 2000b).

*Systems Research, Development, and Integration*

In its 1997 report the Committee on International Science, Engineering, and Technology (CISET) Emerging Infectious Diseases Working Group acknowledged the creation of a DoD Internet-based Central Communications Hub (a GEIS website) as one of the early accomplishments of GEIS. The working group expressed expectations that the site would grow in time to include a private intranet chat line to link the overseas laboratories and a public site that would allow searching of several DoD databases and that would provide the groundwork for the automatic reporting of bacterial resistance patterns and certain reportable diseases (CISET, 1997).

GEIS views GEISWeb as part of its outreach program. It seeks to provide a "one-stop focal point" for the linking of information on infectious diseases from DoD and external parties, but it must do so within the constraints imposed by DoD security and privacy policies (Writer, 2001c). In particular, GEISWeb is designed to (Writer, 2001c):

- promote understanding of GEIS,
- generate an exchange of new ideas and best practices for countering emerging infections,

- provide resource information to health professionals,
- display information about emerging illnesses and broader programmatic issues,
- provide tools for outbreak investigations,
- provide information on training and conferences, and
- provide links to related sites.

The site was redesigned in fiscal year 2001 to improve its usability. GEIS is undertaking a market survey to better identify the needs of DoD and the public (GEIS, 2000b).

## GEIS Program Management

In documents that set the stage for the development of GEIS, it was universally indicated that a central coordinating office for GEIS (a Central Hub) should be established at WRAIR (Bancroft and Schlagel, 1997; CISET, 1997; Zajtchuk, 1995). The Central Hub supports a staff of approximately 13 full- and part-time personnel, including a director and a deputy director and administrative, technical support, and scientific advisory personnel (GEIS, 2001c). The Central Hub is not, however, optimally staffed, according to planning documents (Bancroft and Schlagel, 1997; Cuddy, 1997; Martin, 1997a,b). GEIS has never received the full complement of staff that was intended.

The GEIS Central Hub has access to a flag-level[3] advisory board (Lister, 1997). The GEIS Advisory Board is chaired by DoD (Health Affairs) with membership including the Army, Navy, and Air Force Deputy Surgeons General. Its purview is general oversight of GEIS to include adequacy of staffing, policy and program review, budgetary planning and decisions, and evaluation. Scientific advice is sought from the Armed Forces Epidemiology Board as the need arises. GEIS, through the Central Hub, reports to the Office of the Surgeon General of the U.S. Army (Martin, 1997c). GEIS has no direct command authority over members of its consortium. GEIS is in a period of transition in terms of its position within the organizational structure of the DoD. The IOM committee is aware of efforts to revise GEIS charter documents to improve its linkages within the DoD to position the program to better receive and provide scientific and management guidance (Kelley, 2001c).

The Central Hub's primary role can generally be summarized as coordination and communication. The GEIS Central Hub has further specified description of its duties as follows (Kelley, 2001b):

[3]General officer or admiral rank.

- develop, coordinate, and monitor execution of strategic plan;
- review annual proposals for funding and prioritize support;
- coordinate distribution of funds;
- review and publish annual reports from GEIS-funded agencies;
- assist with obtaining supplementary resources;
- represent GEIS to higher headquarters and other federal, international, and local agencies;
- facilitate CINC-supported civic assistance projects;
- manage public and professional awareness initiatives; and
- foster solutions to emerging infections problems through sponsorship of professional forums.

The GEIS 5-year strategic plan, *Addressing Emerging Infectious Disease Threats: A Strategic Plan for the Department of Defense*, was published in 1998 (GEIS, 1998). The Central Hub also compiles, publishes, and distributes an annual report that documents program progress. Results of GEIS-supported studies are frequently published in the peer-reviewed literature, and select project updates, as well as information on the topic of emerging infections diseases, are posted on GEISWeb.

GEIS project review and the coordination of funding allocations are important tasks of the Central Hub. Such decisions are made by the GEIS director (who is a member of the U.S. Army) and staff (McCarthy, 1998, 1999a,b,c,d,e,f). Both MHS and overseas medical research laboratory activities are chosen for support and receive annual reviews based on the following criteria (GEIS, 2000b; Kelley, 2001b):

- potential to fill a critical gap in MHS public health programs,
- likelihood of triservice or service-wide benefits,
- facilitation of timely public health actions,
- responsiveness to critical operational theater needs,
- accessibility of the nonfiscal resources needed for execution,
- scientific quality,
- whether it is other than an existing core MHS public health program, and
- consistency with the GEIS 5-year strategic plan.

GEIS has also contributed to many professional symposia and professional forums, including the following (Kelley, 2001b):

- International Conference on Emerging Infectious Diseases (1998 and 2000)
- Military Public Health Laboratory Symposium and Workshop, September 21–23, 1999

- Conference and Workshop on Syndromic and Other Surveillance Methods for Emerging Infections, May 23–25, 2000
- Institute of Medicine Forum for Emerging Infectious Disease (ongoing)
- U.S. Medicine Institute-GEIS Forum on Vaccines (March 2001)

Through the Central Hub, GEIS is also represented on many committees, task forces, and related public health decision-making bodies. Among these are CISET, the Asia Pacific Economic Cooperation Office Industrial Science and Technology Working Group, the IOM Infectious Disease Forum, the CDC Overseas Infectious Disease Strategy Review Committee, International Conference on Emerging Infections Planning Committee, Federal Antibiotic Resistance Task Force, the Pan American Health Organization Emerging Infections Task Force, and the WHO Outbreak Response Network Committee (Kelley, 2001b). Additional ties are being pursued with many collaborative agencies. For instance, closer integration with the WHO is being sought through the assignment of a Navy preventive medicine physician to WHO headquarters in Geneva (Kelley, 2001b).

## CONCLUSIONS

GEIS-supported activities within the MHS and the Central Hub constitute a collage of endeavors that, on balance, are consistent with GEIS goals.

Within the MHS and through the Central Hub, GEIS is supporting a number of infectious disease surveillance projects that have the potential to detect emerging infections. These projects encompass GEIS pillar targets, such as drug resistance (e.g., antimalarial drug resistance surveillance, antimicrobial resistance surveillance pilot project, GISP site development), acute febrile illnesses including malaria (e.g., febrile illness surveillance in the Republic of Korea and Uganda, and WRAIR and WHO antimalarial drug resistance surveillance), influenza and respiratory disease (e.g., NHRC triservice surveillance for viral respiratory pathogens, *S. pyogenes*, and antibiotic resistance among *S. pneumoniae* isolates, and the DoD Laboratory-Based Influenza Surveillance Program), and enteric pathogens.

In accordance with its capacity-building goals, GEIS supports the development and maintenance of laboratory capacity within the infrastructure of the MHS. Some of this support is direct (e.g., annual retainer paid directly to USAMRIID). Some capacity building occurs as a by-product of the conduct of GEIS projects. Supporting the development of DoD laboratory centers of excellence for target disease areas can help build capacity valuable to GEIS consortium members and the DoD more generally and can help to encourage linkages within the GEIS consortium. AFIERA and the NHRC, designated centers for influenza and for respiratory disease excellence, respectively, possess laboratory capacity and expertise that have contributed notably to DoD (and U.S.) surveillance and response efforts. Development of additional DoD laboratory centers of excellence that address disease targets that are not well covered within the DoD, such as enteric pathogens, is also worthy of GEIS pursuit. Encouraging laboratories to obtain WHO collaborating center status can increase connections within the public health community by encouraging capacity building and recognition of that capacity.

GEIS has also done an astounding job of leveraging minimal resources to implement capacity-building projects in support of its public health partners overseas. Central Hub-managed efforts to provide training and communications and laboratory resources have been well received and are having tangible results (i.e., in the Caribbean and South America). The GEIS Central Hub has valuable expertise, resources, and linkages to bring to bear in these efforts. However, the committee notes that Central Hub and overseas laboratory capacity-building projects are often conducted separately, at times with little communication or coordination between them. For instance, at the time of subcommittee visits to overseas laboratories, Central Hub capacity-building efforts in Peru were not well coordinated with NMRCD, nor were Central Hub epidemiology training efforts in Kenya and infectious disease surveillance efforts in Uganda coordinated with USAMRU-K. Similarly, although GEIS-supported projects at the 18th MEDCOM in the Republic of Korea do receive some diagnostic support from AFRIMS, these projects are primarily coordinated with the Central Hub and not proximate overseas laboratories (AFRIMS and NAMRU-2). Lack of coordination risks duplication of efforts (e.g., the Central Hub and USAMRU-K have separate plans to implement epidemiology training programs for public health workers in Kenya) and detracts from the development of a cohesive, recognizable program whole.

GEIS, with its triservice focus and coordinating role, can contribute substantially to DoD training activities relevant to emerging infectious disease surveillance and response. The Central Hub-managed Overseas Medical Research Laboratory Orientation Training Program presents valuable opportunities for active-duty junior and midlevel physicians, USUHS students, and other such individuals to gain functional experience. Likewise, this program affords the DoD the opportunity to build an experienced staff base. This program is young, but already at least one individual has indicated that the opportunity to work briefly on a project overseas has solidified his interest in making a long-term commitment to working in an overseas laboratory (Writer, 2001b).

The Overseas Medical Research Laboratory Orientation Training Program represents an important step in achieving GEIS training goals. However, this program, which focuses on the short-term placement of trainees at overseas laboratories, does not fully realize the potential of GEIS to contribute to the training of researchers and public health professionals (DoD personnel and others). Ad hoc training activities are already conducted at many laboratories overseas and within the MHS. By helping to coordinate and promote existing training resources, GEIS may be of benefit to many. GEIS may also wish to consider expanding the Overseas Medical Research Laboratory Orientation Training Program concept, as well as developing additional training programs. For example, programs that would allow MHS public health laboratory personnel[4] to receive epidemic response training at overseas laboratories, programs that place personnel at MHS facilities for specialized laboratory training, and programs that foster increased collaboration with the CDC's Field Epidemiology Training Program (a part of the Training in Epidemiology and Public Health Intervention Network [TEPHINET]) are potential training endeavors that may benefit from and be of benefit to GEIS.

GEIS makes use of other DoD public health surveillance systems, such as DMSS, AFRESS, and others in pursuit of its goals. GEIS also supports the development and implementation of new surveillance systems and techniques, in keeping with its systems research goal. For instance, development of the ESSENCE bioterrorism surveillance system, development of an emerging infectious disease alert component for the new DoD mortality surveillance system, support of the exploratory use of GIS and remote-sensing techniques for surveillance purposes (e.g., surveillance for STDs at Madigan Army Hospital and remote-sensing collaborations with NASA), and many other projects exemplify GEIS's commitment to using new and diverse methods to create a DoD surveillance system that is sensitive to emerging infectious diseases. Many of these efforts show great promise. It is important, however, that GEIS investment in the development of new systems and techniques follows from a clearly established and widely understood need and that large-scale implementation of new systems or techniques follows a thorough evaluation. Competing or redundant systems can adversely affect surveillance and response efforts by consuming valuable resources and by cluttering reporting channels.

The transition that GEIS has made from a concept on paper to a functioning, productive program is in no small way a testament to the indus-

[4]USAMRIID staff representatives, for instance, expressed to the committee an interest in pursuing a training partnership, through GEIS, with the overseas laboratories.

try and ingenuity of Central Hub management. Now that the program has gotten a solid start, it is appropriate to consider whether the program management approaches that helped GEIS take its infant steps are the same approaches that will serve GEIS well in the future. In particular, the Central Hub has, to date, been opportunistically focused on identifying and filling critical gaps in DoD infectious disease surveillance and response capabilities and establishing a base of projects in support of GEIS goals. In doing so, GEIS has amassed an array of projects that, although all valuable in their own right, do not fit together smoothly as part of a cohesive, conspicuous GEIS whole. Coordination and communication, essential program elements and key roles of the Central Hub (Bancroft and Schlagel, 1997; CISET, 1997; GEIS, 1998), are not sufficiently addressed at present.

MHS-based projects can better contribute to GEIS if they are more tightly integrated with each other and are geared toward supporting and complementing surveillance activities conducted in overseas laboratories. MHS laboratories possess valuable diagnostic capabilities and reservoirs of staff expertise. These resources are not put to their highest and best use if their work for GEIS consists primarily of conducting isolated projects.

GEIS would benefit from refinement of the group of MHS-based projects that it funds. The development of a group of core projects that make integrated use of consortium resources, that are sustainable over a lengthy or indefinite time period, and that have the flexibility to address changing surveillance and response needs is preferable to the provision of support for a large number of projects that are relatively narrow in scope, short in duration, and circumspect in their implementation. Scaling back the breadth of GEIS involvement in the MHS may be necessary to develop a group of activities that provide GEIS with improved continuity, congruity, and visibility. The GEIS project review process may need to be revised to accommodate this approach.

At present, Central Hub involvement in the management of projects that it does not directly conduct seems confined largely to the annual review process. For GEIS to function as a program, active management is important. It is important that the management provided by the Central Hub include consistent interaction with staff directing GEIS projects to monitor project progress, identify potential new collaborative activities, and identify needs for assistance. The role of the Central Hub, first and foremost, is to serve as the focal point for GEIS coordination and communication. It is important that other Central Hub activities do not conflict with these tasks.

It is also important that the Central Hub plays an active role in communicating GEIS-generated information within the GEIS consortium, within the DoD, to public health partners, and to the public. Current efforts to disseminate information are noteworthy but insufficient. GEIS can help consortium members develop strategies to share information with public health partners that need the information to take timely action in response to an emerging infectious disease. The Central Hub can also encourage program identity and collaborative activities by routinely collecting GEIS-generated information from consortium members, synthesizing this information as needed, and providing reports back to consortium members and others in a timely fashion.

Tools such as GEISWeb and the DoD Directory of Public Health Laboratory Services can help improve coordination and communication within GEIS and beyond (WHO, 2000a). The concept of a Directory of Public Health Laboratory Services in a system of distributed responsibilities such as the DoD makes good organizational sense. If constructed wisely,[5] the DoD Directory of Public Health Laboratory Services and the broader concept of the Virtual Public Health Laboratory can help make DoD laboratory resources more accessible to GEIS sites and others, encouraging collaboration and use of the full spectrum of DoD laboratory capabilities in the conduct of GEIS projects. GEISWeb also plays a role in fostering communication and the dissemination of information regarding GEIS projects. It may be useful to use GEISWeb as a point of entry into the DoD Directory of Public Health Laboratory Services. These resources cannot, however, take the place of frequent interpersonal communications between Central Hub staff and GEIS project managers at the overseas laboratories and within the MHS.

The committee recognizes that managing a program as diverse and diffuse as GEIS is no small task. It appears to the committee that the Central Hub is limited in its ability to effectively coordinate GEIS by a lack of administrative authority and management resources, including a lack of appropriate staffing (in number and in expertise) and a lack of a clear and consistent means of both receiving and providing scientific and management direction.

## RECOMMENDATIONS

- The GEIS Central Hub needs to be provided with increased administrative authority and management resources to achieve its program management goals.

**Recommendation: Staffing within the Central Hub should be in-**

---

[5]For instance, if it is designed by experienced developers with a specific end product in mind, incorporates input from a clearly defined user group, is flexible enough to accommodate additional modules over time, and is accessible to as wide a user group as appropriate and possible.

**creased so that its communication and coordination responsibilities can be optimally addressed.**

**Recommendation: The Central Hub should have available to it improved means of obtaining more and more frequent management guidance.**

**Recommendation: The Central Hub should be given more management authority so that it can successfully meet its objectives.**

- The infrastructure of the MHS provides an important platform for the support of surveillance for emerging infectious diseases within the nondeployed U.S. military population and for support of the efforts of the overseas medical research laboratories. GEIS investment in MHS public health laboratory activities should focus on developing strong capabilities for identifying and responding to emerging infectious diseases and cultivating collaborative relationships among laboratories so that capabilities are optimally used.

**Recommendation: GEIS projects within the infrastructure of the MHS are important but should be more tightly integrated with each other and better coordinated with and supportive of activities conducted at the overseas laboratories.**

- The development of centers of laboratory excellence within the DoD (e.g., for influenza and respiratory diseases) encourages the availability of specialized capabilities and makes those specialized capabilities more visible within the DoD laboratory system. Additional centers of excellence for underaddressed disease target areas, such as diseases caused by enteric pathogens, should also be grown at appropriate facilities. Similarly, GEIS consortium members should be encouraged to become or to remain WHO Collaborating Centers (e.g., for Emerging Infectious Diseases), as this promotes capacity and recognition of that capacity.

**Recommendation: GEIS efforts to build MHS public health laboratory capacity to detect and respond to emerging infectious diseases should be clearly focused and should be increased.**

- The research and development that GEIS supports in the context of information technology and laboratory diagnostics should be limited to those areas for which other expertise and venues do not exist. Exploration of new surveillance techniques and methodologies, such as syndromic surveillance, are also important but should be scientifically validated before they become widely enmeshed in GEIS. Communications tools, such as GEISWeb and the Directory of Public Health Laboratory Services-Virtual Public Health Laboratory can be very valuable to GEIS and need to be rigorously planned, and produced and maintained by developers possessing extensive expertise and experience.

**Recommendation: The development of new systems resources is an important goal of GEIS, but the needs and specifications for innovative surveillance systems should be clearly defined before they are undertaken, and caution should be used when implementing unproven systems on a large scale.**

• Current efforts to provide training and communications and laboratory resources to public health partners are producing tangible benefits, but insufficient coordination within GEIS detracts from the effectiveness and recognition of these efforts.

**Recommendation: Central Hub-managed international capacity-building projects should be better coordinated with DoD laboratory facilities overseas and within the MHS, as appropriate.**

• GEIS can contribute substantially to DoD training activities relevant to emerging infectious disease surveillance and response. The Overseas Medical Research Laboratory Orientation Training Program and other ad hoc training activities currently in place are noteworthy and important, but additional GEIS involvement in the training of research and public health professionals—including, but not limited to, DoD personnel—can make existing training activities more efficient, productive, and visible and can help encourage the development of additional training programs.

**Recommendation: Central Hub involvement in coordinating and supporting training activities relevant to emerging infectious disease surveillance and response should be increased.**

• The Central Hub needs to increase its efforts to provide centralized coordination and scientific direction for GEIS projects. Projects should be better coordinated among members of the GEIS consortium. Project progress would also benefit from more and more frequent scientific guidance.

**Recommendation: The GEIS Central Hub should**

**Provide clear and specific guidance to laboratories regarding the goals of GEIS and the qualities that GEIS projects are expected to possess, actively assist laboratories in developing project plans, and provide periodic scientific guidance for projects under way, as needed.**

**Provide a mechanism for project review that is structured, that is clearly and consistently defined, that allows adequate time for**

**project conduct between reviews, that results in timely feedback to the laboratories proposing projects, and that is carried out by a diverse panel of experts including Central Hub staff and others, such as senior DoD laboratory staff, Military Infectious Disease Research Program (MIDRP) staff, and other DoD and non-DoD representatives.**

**Consistently interact with staff directing GEIS projects to monitor project progress, evolving potential for collaboration, and needs for assistance.**

- It is important that projects be directed by regionally appropriate overseas and MHS-based laboratories.

**Recommendation: Given personnel and other resource shortages, Central Hub conduct of surveillance projects is undesirable and should be minimized and avoided to the extent possible.**

- At present GEIS does not regularly produce or distribute an informational product that synthesizes data from its consortium members and that feeds the information back to its consortium members and other users in a timely manner.

**Recommendation: Improved means of centrally collecting, analyzing (as appropriate), and distributing surveillance data and other information in a timely manner should be developed and implemented.**

## AGENDAS

### IOM and DoD-GEIS MHS Program Review
### San Diego, California
### January 9–10, 2001

*Tuesday, January 9, 2001*

| | |
|---|---|
| 0800-0815 | **Welcome/Introductory Remarks**<br>CAPT T. Contreras, NHRC Commanding Officer<br>Dr. Berkelman, Acting Chair |
| 0815-0845 | **Orientation to GEIS the MHS**<br>COL Kelley |
| 0845-1000 | **Review of Air Force Central Hub Activities**<br>LTC Neville |
| 1000-1015 | Break |
| 1015-1300 | **Review of NHRC Activities**<br>LCDR Ryan and CAPT Gray and Staff |

| | |
|---|---|
| 1300-1345 | Lunch at NHRC |
| 1345-1415 | **Tour of NHRC GEIS**<br>CAPT Gray |
| 1415-1500 | **Travel to NEPMU** |
| 1500-1525 | **Review of NEHC GEIS Activities**<br>CDR Murphy |
| 1525-1545 | **Review of NEPMU GEIS Activities**<br>CDR Thornton |
| 1545-1605 | **Tour of NEPMU**<br>CAPT Tueller |
| 1605-1635 | Travel to Naval Hospital, San Diego |
| 1635-1710 | **Presentation on Antibiotic Resistance Surveillance**<br>CAPT Davis |
| 1710-1800 | Naval hospital laboratory and questions for and laboratory staff on laboratory-based surveillance for reportable infections and antibiotic resistance |
| 1900 | Dinner for presenters and IOM committee members |

*Wednesday, January 10, 2001 (at NHRC)*

| | |
|---|---|
| 0800-0845 | **ESSENCE, and Syndromic Surveillance**<br>MAJ Pavlin |
| 0845-0910 | **Madigan STD Project**<br>COL Gunzenhauser |
| 0910-0940 | **Korea Malaria Surveillance**<br>MAJ Pavlin and LTC Klein |
| 0940-1010 | **Uganda Projects**<br>MAJ Pavlin |
| 1010-1100 | Follow-questions and discussions |
| 1100 | IOM committee members to return to hotel for working session |

**Fifth Meeting of the Institute of Medicine Committee to Review the Department of Defense Global Emerging Infections Surveillance and Response System**
**Washington, DC**
**6[6], 7, 8 March 2001**

*Tuesday, March 6, 2001: Site Visit, Ft. Detrick, Maryland*

| | |
|---|---|
| 1330-1400 | **USAMRIID briefing**<br>COL Ted Cieslak and Dr. George Ludwig |

[6]Supplemental session, not all committee members present.

| | |
|---|---|
| 1400-1445 | **USAMRIID diagnostics**<br>Dr. George Ludwig |
| 1445-1530 | **Tour of USAMRIID**<br>COL Ted Cieslak |
| 1530-1630 | **Discussion with MIDRP**<br>COL Charles Hoke |
| 1630-1700 | **Discussion with MRMC Command Group**<br>COL John Glenn |

*Wednesday, March 7, 2001*

| | |
|---|---|
| 0800-0805 | **Welcome and introductions**<br>Dr. Philip Brachman |
| 0805-0845 | **AFIP Virtual Public Health Laboratory**<br>Dr. Joel Gaydos and Dr. Victor Kalasinsky |
| 0845-0915 | **AFIP Mortality Surveillance Project**<br>Dr. Joel Gaydos |
| 0915-1030 | **Overview of Other DoD Surveillance**<br>COL Patrick Kelley |
| 1030-1100 | **Collaborations with NASA**<br>LTC Kenneth Linthicum |
| 1100-1200 | **Other Activities of GEIS Central Hub**<br>(OCONUS training, Humanitarian assistance, Website)<br>Mr. James Writer |
| 1200-1300 | Catered lunch at IOM |
| 1300-1400 | **Other activities of GEIS Central Hub continued (Management, External Relations)**<br>COL Patrick Kelley |
| 1400-1500 | Follow-up discussions with presenters and invited collaborators |
| 1500-1700 | Closed session |
| 1700 | Adjournment |

*Thursday, March 8, 2001*

| | |
|---|---|
| 0800-1500 | IOM committee meets in closed session |

## GEIS CENTRAL HUB AND MILITARY HEALTH SYSTEM ACTIVITIES REVIEW: MEETING PARTICIPANTS, GUESTS, AND OTHER CONTRIBUTORS

Assaf Anyamba, Goddard Space Flight Center, NASA, Greenbelt, Maryland

Carolyn Baker, Naval Health Research Center, San Diego, California
Linda Canas, Diagnostic Virology, Brooks Air Force Base, San Antonio, Texas
Theodore J. Cieslak, Operational Medicine Department, U.S. Army Medical Research Institute of Infectious Diseases, Ft. Detrick, Maryland
T. Contreras, Naval Health Research Center, San Diego, California
Jonathan Davis, Institute of Medicine, Washington, District of Columbia
Susan R. Davis, Department of Defense Global Emerging Infections Surveillance and Response System, Division of Preventive Medicine, Walter Reed Army Institute of Research, Silver Spring, Maryland
Matthew DiFranco, collaborator, Naval Health Research Center respiratory disease surveillance projects, San Diego, California
Benedict Diniega, Chemical and Biological Defense Health Affairs, U.S. Department of Defense, Washington, District of Columbia
Maria Gabriela Fernandez-DiFranco, Naval Health Research Center, San Diego, California
Joel Gaydos, Department of Defense Global Emerging Infections Surveillance and Response System, Division of Preventive Medicine, Walter Reed Army Institute of Research, Silver Spring, Maryland
Michele Ginsberg, San Diego County Health Department, San Diego, California
John Frazier Glenn, Medical Research and Materiel Command, Ft. Detrick, Maryland
Greg Gray, Naval Health Research Center, San Diego, California
Jeffrey Gunzenhauser, Public Health Residency, Madigan Army Medical Center, Tacoma, Washington
Tony Hawksworth, Naval Health Research Center, San Diego, California
Charles Hoke, Military Infectious Disease Research Program, U.S. Army Medical Research and Materiel Command, Ft. Detrick, Maryland
Marie Hudspeth, Naval Health Research Center, San Diego, California
Victor F. Kalasinsky, Armed Forces Institute of Pathology, Washington, District of Columbia
Patrick Kelley, Department of Defense Global Emerging Infections Surveillance and Response System, Division of Preventive Medicine, Walter Reed Army Institute of Research, Silver Spring, Maryland
Terry A. Klein, 18th Medical Command, Republic of Korea
Kenneth Linthicum, Department of Defense Global Emerging Infections Surveillance and Response System, Division of Preventive

Medicine, Walter Reed Army Institute of Research, Silver Spring, Maryland
George V. Ludwig, Applied Diagnostics Branch, U.S. Army Medical Research Institute of Infectious Diseases, Ft. Detrick, Maryland
Victor MacIntosh, Preventive Medicine Division, Air Force Medical Operations Agency
Marrietta Malasig, Naval Health Research Center, San Diego, California
AbuBakr Marzouk, Office of the Air Force Medical Examiner, Armed Forces Institute of Pathology, Washington, District of Columbia
Michael McCarthy, Department of Defense Global Emerging Infections Surveillance and Response System, Division of Preventive Medicine, Walter Reed Army Institute of Research, Silver Spring, Maryland
Jamie McKeehan, Naval Health Research Center, San Diego, California
Wilbur K. Milhous, Experimental Therapeutics, Walter Reed Army Institute of Research, Silver Spring, Maryland
Melinda Moore, Office of International and Refugee Health, Office of Public Health and Science, Office of the Secretary, U.S. Department of Health and Human Services, Rockville, Maryland
Brian P. Murphy, Preventive Medicine, Navy Environmental Health Center, Norfolk, Virginia
James Neville, Force Health Protection and Surveillance Branch, Brooks Air Force Base, San Antonio, Texas
Matt O'Shea, Naval Health Research Center, San Diego, California
Lawrence Palinkas, Division of Family and Preventive Medicine, University of California, San Diego, California
John S. Parker, U.S. Army Medical Research and Materiel Command, Ft. Detrick, Maryland
Julie Pavlin, Department of Defense Global Emerging Infections Surveillance and Response System, Division of Preventive Medicine, Walter Reed Army Institute of Research, Silver Spring, Maryland
Saibal Poddar, Naval Health Research Center, San Diego, California
Bob Potter, Office of the Air Force Medical Examiner, Armed Forces Institute of Pathology, Washington, District of Columbia
Margaret Ryan, Naval Health Research Center, San Diego, California
Paul Sato, Naval Health Research Center, San Diego, California
Lori Senini, San Diego County Border Health, San Diego, California
Dawn Taggett, Naval Health Research Center, San Diego, California
Scott Thornton, Navy Evironmental and Preventive Medicine Unit Number 5, San Diego, California
John Tueller, Navy Evironmental and Preventive Medicine Unit Number 5, San Diego, California

James Writer, Department of Defense Global Emerging Infections Surveillance and Response System, Division of Preventive Medicine, Walter Reed Army Institute of Research, Silver Spring, Maryland

# 8

# Summary Conclusions and Recommendations

## SUMMARY CONCLUSIONS

### GEIS in Concept

The development of the Global Emerging Infections Surveillance and Response System (GEIS) is, conceptually, an appropriate U.S. Department of Defense (DoD) response to Presidential Decision Directive NSTC-7 (NSTC, 1996) and to the concerns and recommendations expressed in the 1992 Institute of Medicine (IOM) report *Emerging Infections: Microbial Threats to Health in the United States.*

GEIS goals, as outlined in the GEIS strategic plan, address the areas of mission expansion that NSTC-7 mandates. GEIS provides a means of coordinating DoD efforts to address "global surveillance, training, research, and response to emerging infectious disease threats" (NSTC, 1996, p. 4), as directed. GEIS also possesses the components necessary to be consistent with IOM guidance regarding the essential elements of an effective global surveillance network, including the following (IOM, 1992, p. 6):

1. a mechanism for detecting (using clinical presentation as the criterion) clusters of new or unusual diseases or syndromes;

2. laboratories capable of identifying and characterizing infectious agents;

3. an information system to analyze reportable occurrences and disseminate summary data; and

4. a response mechanism to provide feedback to reporting agencies and individuals and, if necessary, to mobilize investigative and control efforts of local and international agencies.

Overseas laboratories, the military health system (MHS) infrastructure, and the GEIS Central Hub provide the basic framework necessary for GEIS to conform to this ideal type. Because GEIS supports activities at DoD overseas laboratories, it is also, in a sense, responsive to IOM recommendations calling for sustained support of these resources (IOM, 1992).

## GEIS in Context

*Within the DoD*

GEIS is a new mission that has been added to operations carried out at existing DoD facilities within the United States and abroad. GEIS does not and cannot sustain these facilities alone. The success of GEIS is predicated on the availability of resources at overseas research laboratories and supporting MHS capabilities sufficient to maintain an appropriate base for GEIS operations. DoD laboratory resources, particularly overseas medical research laboratories, have been and continue to be imperiled.

In 1992, the IOM noted that (IOM, 1992, p. 149):

> The [Committee on Emerging Microbial Threats to Health] is concerned that some of these [DoD overseas medical research] laboratories have been closed in the past, for reasons related both to insufficient funding and changes in mission priorities, and that further closings could jeopardize the United States' ability to detect and respond to emerging infectious disease threats.

A new DoD research facility, the ninth largest biomedical research facility in the country, was recently completed in Maryland (Walter Reed Army Institute of Research, 1998). The facility houses Army and Navy medical research and development command headquarters, as well as the GEIS Central Hub. This facility is an outstanding resource domestically. It reflects an important investment in DoD laboratory infrastructure. Other DoD laboratories are also in need of revitalization. GEIS would benefit from increased capacity within existing laboratories and the introduction of additional DoD laboratories overseas, particularly in areas of high biodiversity and other locations where the potential for the emergence of infectious diseases is high. At a minimum, it is important to GEIS that existing laboratory facilities be maintained.

At the time of preparation of the 1992 IOM report, seven overseas laboratories were in existence (IOM, 1992). By the time that Presidential Decision Directive NSTC-7 was released in 1996, there were six laboratories. At the time of this review, five overseas laboratories remain. Domestic capabilities have also been curtailed through the closure of the Letterman Army Institute of Research (GEIS, 1998). This is a discouraging trend that does not favor the success of GEIS. *Loss of laboratory infrastructure, particularly overseas, limits the DoD's global emerging infectious disease surveillance and response capacity and, accordingly, GEIS prospects.*

At some DoD laboratories, in the United States and overseas, the committee noted a lack of full integration between DoD research and infectious disease surveillance priorities. Establishing GEIS within the existing framework of the DoD laboratories can benefit the research and infectious disease surveillance missions of the DoD, respectively. GEIS can benefit from the scientific and technical facilities, staff expertise, established research efforts, and working relationships already in existence. In return, GEIS can strengthen and build partnerships and can provide surveillance information useful in guiding the development of future research projects, maximizing benefits to the U.S. military. Finding a balance between these missions is important to the success of both. Each mission is critically important and is essential to national security. The observed discontinuity benefits neither and harms both. *If GEIS is to be of optimal benefit, its mission will need to be fully understood, accepted, and balanced against the needs and resources of other DoD laboratory stakeholders.*

GEIS is not optimally positioned to receive or provide direction, which weakens its effectiveness overall. Clear and consistent channels for reporting GEIS information to higher command authorities are also not sufficiently defined. *It is important that GEIS management authority is commensurate with GEIS management responsibility if the information that GEIS generates is to result in timely action.*

### *National Partners*

The DoD is one of several U.S. government agencies that have a significant interest in, and responsibility for, addressing emerging infectious diseases. Each agency brings to the table important resources and certain limitations, and each fills a particular niche. The DoD, for its part, possesses unique laboratory capabilities, many situated in diverse forward locations, and has a vested interest in addressing emerging infectious diseases as a matter of national security (NIC, 2000).

The relationship between the Centers for Disease Control and Prevention (CDC) and the DoD is an important one and warrants particular attention. The DoD and the CDC have, in the past, provided each other with backup support and entered into collaborative relationships on an as-needed basis. Recent changes in the missions of both the CDC and the DoD are bringing their respective program interests and spheres of operation into increasingly close contact. Through GEIS, the DoD has expanded its role overseas to include emerging infectious disease surveillance, response, and training and capacity building (GEIS, 1998). Conversely, the CDC has recently developed a global infectious disease strategy that formalizes CDC interests and operations in emerging infectious diseases internationally and increases its research presence (Dowell, 2001). The committee is aware that the CDC plans to locate its first international surveillance program in Thailand and is considering the development of a site in Kenya as well. GEIS is active in both Thailand and Kenya.

The CDC's new global strategy for addressing emerging infectious diseases identifies six priority areas: international outbreak assistance, support of a global approach to disease surveillance, applied research on diseases of global importance, application of proven public health tools, and public health training and capacity building (Dowell, 2001). *CDC and DoD GEIS strategies for addressing emerging infectious diseases reflect very similar goals, related infectious disease target areas, and overlapping arenas of operation. As these activites evolve, collaboration between the CDC and the DoD—at the management level, as well as in the field—will be of utmost importance if both are to make efficient and effective use of limited resources.*

*International Partnerships*

Addressing emerging infectious diseases is an issue of global importance and shared responsibility. The GEIS strategic plan (GEIS, 1998) calls for collaboration with other international partners, such as the World Health Organization (WHO), and governmental agencies in foreign countries, such as ministries of health. The WHO, in particular, is the focal point for communicable disease control efforts worldwide, and it recognizes the need for "collaboration between WHO and all potential technical partners in the area of epidemic alert and response, including relevant public sectors, intergovernmental organizations, nongovernmental organizations, and the private sector" (WHO, 2001a, p.1). The DoD, specifically GEIS, is considered to be such a partner (WHO, 1998). Many, but not all, members of the GEIS consortium—DoD partners in GEIS—are or are seeking to become WHO collaborating centers. WHO collaborating centers are an important part of the WHO "network of networks," through which technical backup, research, training, and transfer of technology are directed to support disease surveillance and control efforts (WHO, 1996). It has been noted that incorporation of DoD laboratories into this network would be of benefit to global infectious disease surveillance efforts (D'Amelio and Heymann, 1998). *The committee agrees that WHO Collaborating Center for Emerging Infectious Diseases and other WHO collaborating center status is in keeping with the intent of NSTC-7 (NSTC, 1996), GEIS goals (GEIS, 1998), and U.S. and international interests.*

## GEIS in Practice

Having reviewed the implementation of GEIS at the overseas laboratories, within the infrastructure of the MHS, and within the GEIS Central Hub, the committee concludes the following regarding GEIS as a whole:

### *Surveillance*

*The committee concludes that the GEIS pillars are reasonable targets for emerging infectious disease surveillance, given available resources and the partners and stakeholders to whom GEIS is responsible. Current GEIS pillar areas are generally being well addressed by GEIS, primarily through activities at the overseas laboratories, but also through activities within the infrastructure of the MHS and through the Central Hub.* The committee is concerned, however, that the existing pillar structure is incompletely defined and understood. GEIS pillars are interpreted somewhat differently and acted upon somewhat differently at each of the overseas laboratories (see Chapters 2 to 7). Presentation of the pillar concept within the GEIS strategic plan (GEIS, 1998) is vague. Rigid adherence to a pillar construct can impinge upon the responsiveness of GEIS to regionally relevant emerging infectious disease threats. The committee notes, for instance, that disease areas of global importance, such as tuberculosis, are absent from the current GEIS pillar structure and are underaddressed within GEIS, even though host countries identify them as priorities. On the other hand, lack of structure can result in fragmented, inefficient activities that render GEIS ineffective as a program. It is important to the success of GEIS that the parameters and the intent of the pillar concept be clear to consortium members and partners alike.

### *Systems Research, Development, and Integration*

> [GEIS will] develop the information management tools for clinicians, laboratorians, pathologists, epidemiologists, and preventive medicine/ public health practitioners to address the unique aspects and concepts of emerging infectious disease detection and prevention (GEIS, 1998, p. 28).

GEIS is actively involved in the development and implementation of new surveillance-related systems and in devising new components and uses for existing systems. Many of these developments show great promise (e.g., the DoD Directory of Public Health Laboratory Services, Early Warning Outbreak Response System, Electronic Surveillance System for the Early Notification of Community-Based Epidemics, and numerous others). It is important, however, that the needs and specifications for innovative systems be clearly defined before they are undertaken and that caution be used when implementing unproven systems on a large-scale basis.

*Response*

> A surveillance network must do more than detect cases of disease. It must also collect data on those cases, analyze them in some useful fashion, and disseminate the findings of the analyses to people who can use the information. Surveillance alone, however, is insufficient to address emerging infectious disease adequately. A response mechanism is necessary as well (IOM, 1992, p. 135).

> The missions, capabilities, roles, and priorities of all key organizations must be known and understood to accomplish effective, efficient communication and coordination. All key organizations must be in agreement to enable coordinated, timely, and appropriate responses to emerging infections (GEIS, 1998, p. 38).

DoD overseas laboratories have historically been active in responding to emerging infectious disease epidemics, typically in response to the request of host-country governments or partner agencies. *The mandate and the resources provided by GEIS benefit DoD epidemic response efforts.*

> [GEIS will] improve rapid response capability and coordinated contingency plans for the emergence of new strains of known pathogens, particularly influenza, that threaten to cause pandemic disease (GEIS, 1998, p. 34).

> [GEIS will] develop and successfully staff a DoD assessment and response plan for military medical treatment facilities and DoD beneficiary populations (GEIS, 1998, p. 36).

> [GEIS will] develop and successfully staff a DoD assessment and response plan for a US military emerging infections response in a foreign country (GEIS, 1998, p. 36).

*GEIS has also contributed to the development of epidemic response capacity through the development of new systems, system components, and strategies* (e.g., by fostering the Air Force Institute for Environmental Safety and Occupational Health Risk Analysis influenza alert component). GEIS does not, however, appear to have actively pursued the development of formal, laboratory-specific response plans to guide laboratories, particularly overseas laboratories, in managing requests for assistance.

> [GEIS will] enhance the prompt implementation of all prevention and control strategies for emerging infections to include improving communication about emerging agents (GEIS, 1998, p. 35).

In addition to supporting responses to epidemics, as part of its efforts to respond to the threat of emerging infectious diseases, GEIS has conducted studies and prepared presentations and publications that document emerging infectious disease problems and that develop awareness of these problems. GEIS has also developed and recommended solutions and fostered the implementation and evaluation of interventions (e.g., for sexually transmitted diseases) aimed at preventing and controlling infectious diseases. *The committee concludes that GEIS has generally contributed to national and international knowledge of emerging and reemerging infectious diseases as the result of these efforts.*

### *Training and Capacity Building*

> The laboratories are…a vital source for recruiting and training laboratory personnel for the U.S. military (IOM, 1992, p. 149).

> DoD will make available its overseas laboratory facilities, as appropriate, to serve as focal points for training of foreign technicians and epidemiologists (NSTC, 1996, p. 5).

> [GEIS will] support programs and efforts, including residency training, to ensure the ready availability of the professional expertise and support personnel needed to better understand, monitor, control, and prevent emerging infections (GEIS, 1998, p. 37).

GEIS supports training indirectly by supporting laboratories that in turn support their own distinct training activities. Through the Central Hub, GEIS has also implemented the Overseas Medical Research Laboratory Orientation Training Program, a resource for training DoD preventive medicine personnel, and is also providing training to foreign national public health professionals as part of its capacity-building efforts (e.g., it is providing training in laboratory information systems, computer use, and epidemiology). Additional opportunities exist to work more closely with GEIS consortium members, including the U.S. Army Medical Research Institute of Infectious Diseases (USAMRIID), as well as with public health partners and academic institutions to further address DoD training needs. *The committee concludes that current GEIS efforts to address training needs are laudable, but are modest relative to the needs of the DoD and its partners and to the potential contributions of GEIS.*

> One of the biggest potential barriers to the implementation of a global surveillance network is the transfer of information from and to remote sites in many developing countries that have inadequate telecommunications capabilities (IOM, 1992, pp. 134–135).

> [GEIS will] conduct humanitarian assistance projects in conjunction with the CINC [commander in chief, unified combatant command] Overseas, Humanitarian, Disaster, and Civil AID Program (OHDACA) (GEIS, 1998, p. 38).

GEIS, through activities at the overseas laboratories and the Central Hub and with the support of the unified combatant commands, has done a noteworthy job of assisting with the development of laboratory and communications infrastructures within partner countries. *Current GEIS efforts to build the capacity of its public health partners through the provision of training and support of laboratory and communications infrastructures are having beneficial effects.*

> DoD will ensure the availability of diagnostic capacity at its [domestic and overseas laboratories] using existing DoD resources (NSTC, 1996, p. 5).

GEIS is building capacity within the DoD by supporting the development and maintenance of laboratory diagnostic capacity directly (e.g., through funding of USAMRIID's diagnostic capability) and indirectly (e.g., through funding of projects that result in the development of laboratory infrastructure). *Sustaining and expanding DoD laboratory diagnostic capacity is an important activity that is in GEIS's interests and that could be better and more directly addressed.*

#### *Other Considerations*

The committee also identified a number of factors that are of crosscutting, paramount importance to GEIS and that are therefore discussed separately below.

### *Staffing*

> If necessary, DoD will seek Chief of Mission concurrence to raise personnel ceilings at overseas laboratories (NSTC, 1996, p. 5).

> DoD's recent demand for epidemiologists...has resulted in a shortage recognized by the Army Personnel Command of roughly 50 preventive medicine physicians. In the overseas arena, although DoD labs have highly expert scientists and lab capabilities, their number is grossly insufficient to have a regional impact unless training of local scientists is implemented as a form of leveraging (GEIS, 1998, p. 37).

*The committee concludes that additional staffing is needed to support GEIS,* particularly at the overseas laboratories, but within the Central Hub as well. Personnel at overseas laboratories have been added as the result of GEIS, but GEIS does not have the full complement of staff that was intended (Bancroft and Schlagel, 1997; Cuddy, 1997; Martin, 1997a,b). GEIS implementation has been adversely affected by this lack of staffing.

In particular, insufficient numbers of personnel possessing applied epidemiological knowledge are available to guide surveillance activities.

Also, additional staffing is needed to effectively coordinate the training needs of DoD personnel, foreign national public health workers, and others. GEIS would also benefit from having additional project management staff available within the laboratories and the Central Hub.

Presidential Decision Directive NSTC-7 explicitly recognizes that GEIS brings with it increased staffing needs. Personnel ceilings are, however, only one obstacle affecting GEIS staffing: there are simply not enough qualified DoD personnel available to fill vacancies. *GEIS is pursuing training, the hiring of foreign service nationals, and the assignment of CDC staff to meet staffing needs. All of these approaches are appropriate and important and could be expanded and more actively pursued to meet staffing needs.*

### *Communication*

> A surveillance network must do more than detect cases of disease. It must also collect data on those cases, analyze them in some useful fashion, and disseminate the findings of the analyses to people who can use the information (IOM, 1992, p. 135).
>
> [GEIS will] disseminate aggregate laboratory information about emerging infections and antimicrobial resistance obtained from DoD medical facilities worldwide to all DoD laboratories, hospitals, and practicing physicians (GEIS, 1998, p. 35).
>
> [GEIS will] use diverse communication methods for wider and more effective delivery of critical public health information, alert messages, and prevention and control recommendations (GEIS, 1998, p. 35).
>
> [GEIS will] establish mechanisms for timely and systematic exchanges of surveillance information and laboratory specimens among public health agencies of different countries, the CDC, WHO, and DoD (GEIS, 1998, p. 20).
>
> The CISET [Committee on International Science, Engineering, and Technology] subcommittee on quarantine and containment stated in its recommendations that surveillance data on military populations should be exchanged with relevant state health authorities to ensure that disease importations are properly managed not only within the DoD but also with respect to affected civilian populations (GEIS, 1998, p. 18).

*Current GEIS efforts to communicate surveillance and other information within the GEIS consortium, within the DoD, to public health partners, and to the public are noteworthy but insufficient.* It is of particular importance that mechanisms exist for the rapid and effective communication of information to public health partners who are positioned to take response action, such as U.S. partner agencies, international organizations, and ministries of health. At present, strategies for sharing information with public health partners have not been formally developed, although in many cases good practices have evolved. The committee recognizes that the methods and needs for the sharing of data vary greatly within the GEIS consortium, but it concludes that it is important that these needs be assessed and that communication channels be identified and opened.

It is also important for the GEIS Central Hub to collect surveillance data and other information from consortium members in a systematic, timely manner, analyze this information as appropriate, and report this information back to consortium members and other relevant DoD personnel, public health partners, and the public. Current GEIS information dissemination efforts include production of annual reports, publication of study results in the peer-reviewed literature, presentation of GEIS information at meetings and conferences, periodic publication of laboratory newsletters and updates, and posting of periodic updates on the GEIS website (GEISWeb). Current information dissemination efforts are diverse and important, but they do not constitute a cohesive, regular GEIS product.

### *Coordination and Collaboration*

> To be effective, any global infectious disease surveillance network must be interactive and reciprocal. It is especially important that U.S.-funded laboratories engaged in infectious disease surveillance in foreign countries operate in partnership with host-country facilities (IOM, 1992, p. 134).
>
> [GEIS will] ensure that DoD surveillance systems complement and support local, regional, national, and international surveillance efforts (GEIS, 1998, p. 17).
>
> [GEIS will] develop and maintain coordination and communications systems among clinicians, pathologists, laboratory personnel, preventive medicine personnel, researchers, DoD medical executives, and other DoD parties and external agencies to achieve an integrated GEIS (GEIS, 1998, p. 15).

*GEIS is actively fostering collaboration and coordination with international partners and governmental agencies in partner countries.* This is important to ensure that GEIS projects complement and support other efforts. A DoD preventive medicine physician has been assigned through GEIS to work at WHO headquarters in Geneva, Switzerland. This sharing of staff benefits the DoD and GEIS by increasing awareness of GEIS within the public health community and by fostering the exchange of ideas. Additional steps, such as encouraging consortium members to seek WHO collaborating center status, can benefit the coordination and support of GEIS projects internationally. When engaging international partners, it is important that GEIS present a unified program front; that is to say, the Central Hub and overseas laboratory staff need to closely coordinate planning and implementation of all GEIS activities.

*GEIS is taking important steps to strengthen collaborations with U.S. partner agencies, but more needs to be done to formalize these partnerships.* GEIS notes that the establishment of interagency agreements, for instance, with the CDC and the State Department, is a high priority (GEIS, 1998). Other potential partners, such as the U.S. Agency for International Development (USAID), have yet to fully realize the potential value that collaboration with GEIS can bring, and these partnerships are also worthy of vigorous pursuit. The committee agrees that formalizing and strengthening these relationships is important to the success of GEIS and, more generally, U.S. efforts to address emerging infectious diseases.

*GEIS has also done a noteworthy job of making use of existing DoD capabilities.* Unified combatant command capabilities and resources have contributed greatly to GEIS. GEIS is also mindful of separate DoD public health surveillance activities (e.g., the Defense Medical Surveillance System, the Naval Disease Reporting System, the Shipboard Non-Tactical ADP [automated data processor] Automated Medical System, and the Air Force Reportable Events Surveillance System) in the conduct of its work.

*The current level of collaboration between overseas and MHS laboratories and between those members of GEIS and the GEIS Central Hub could be improved.* To limit redundancy among GEIS projects, to leverage limited resources, and to ensure that the respective parts of GEIS function together as a whole, it is important that laboratory activities be well coordinated and that these activities be collaborative whenever possible. This not only includes collaboration among overseas laboratories with similar regional interests but also necessitates increased coordination among GEIS MHS-based activities and an increased focus of MHS activities and the MHS laboratory infrastructure in support of overseas laboratory surveillance efforts. It is important that the primary occupation of the Central Hub be the active coordination and guidance of projects carried out within MHS and overseas laboratories.

Tools such as GEISWeb and the DoD Directory of Public Health Laboratory Services can improve means of interaction and can encourage collaboration. Also, at many facilities within the GEIS consortium, a dedicated program manager has been assigned to GEIS. This approach seems to benefit coordination of GEIS projects.

### Evaluation

Regular, scientific- and management-related guidance and periodic program review are important at the GEIS management level. *It is essential that GEIS management (i.e., the Central Hub) has available to it clear, appropriate means of routinely receiving authoritative, timely scientific and man-*

*agement guidance. It is also important that GEIS be subject to periodic external review to determine whether the goals of GEIS are being addressed and whether those goals remain appropriate.* On the basis of conversations with and documentation received from laboratory staff (Kelley, 2001c), it does not appear to the committee that the current mechanisms of providing direction to the GEIS Central Hub are sufficient.

*Routine, standardized review of GEIS projects is important.* At present, GEIS projects are reviewed annually by a small number of Central Hub staff. GEIS may benefit from a broader, more standardized review process (including use of structured proposal guidelines and timelines) and expansion of the panel of reviewers to include non-Central Hub staff, such as representatives from partner agencies, overseas and MHS laboratory personnel, and other DoD representatives (e.g., Military Infectious Disease Research Program staff). It may also be useful to lengthen the project approval and funding cycle to allow projects to mature and to allow improved planning of new projects, between reviews.

> [GEIS will] evaluate the effectiveness and economic benefit of existing and proposed strategies to detect and prevent emerging infections (GEIS, 1998, p. 29).

*It is important that the need for new systems and methodologies is assessed and the value of prototype systems is established before large GEIS investments are made in their development or use.* GEIS is investing, according to its goals, in the development and introduction of a number of new surveillance-related systems and methodologies. It is important that GEIS thoroughly evaluate the need for new systems; thoroughly plan system development, including the identification of systems developers with extensive relevant expertise and experience; and evaluate prototype systems to ensure that they are structured to optimally contribute to GEIS.

## SUMMARY RECOMMENDATIONS

• GEIS is a critical and unique resource for the United States in the context of global affairs. It is the only U.S. entity that is devoted to infectious diseases globally and that has broad-based laboratory capacities in overseas settings. GEIS goals, as outlined in its strategic plan, *Addressing Emerging Infectious Disease Threats: A Strategic Plan for the Department of Defense* (GEIS, 1998), address the areas of mission expansion that NSTC-7 mandates (NSTC, 1996). GEIS has the potential to meet and even exceed the expectations of Presidential Decision Directive NSTC-7 in its implementation. To date, significant progress has been made toward meeting the goals of the program. The committee notes that investment in GEIS is small compared to the challenge of emerging infectious diseases. Consideration should be given to increasing DoD investment in GEIS to a level at which GEIS can have a more substantial impact internationally. The GEIS budget is quite small compared to the budgets of those agencies and programs with which GEIS seeks to partner.

It is important, however, to keep in mind that GEIS was created by appending programmatic requirements onto existing DoD bases of operation. The continued success of GEIS is predicated on the availability of resources, through GEIS and others, sufficient to support the facilities that host GEIS and on the ability of those facilities to balance the demands of multiple stakeholders. Research and public health surveillance missions are of critical importance to the DoD and are essential to national security. Emerging infectious disease surveillance is an important part of DoD capacity to assess potential threats to the health of U.S. forces. Research and public health surveillance missions can be balanced so that they are mutually beneficial.

GEIS would also benefit from the expansion of the DoD facilities available to support it. Increased capacity within existing facilities and creation of additional laboratories in areas of high biodiversity and in other regions of the world where there is strong potential for infectious diseases to emerge would benefit GEIS surveillance efforts. The committee recognizes that to respond to the recommendations in this report and to fulfill the mission of the GEIS program, a considerable increase in funding and personnel resources will be required.

**Recommendation: Support for GEIS and the facilities that sustain it should be increased to allow GEIS to completely fulfill its potential.**

• If GEIS is to be of optimal benefit, its mission will need to be fully understood, accepted, and balanced against the needs and resources of other DoD laboratory stakeholders. To work in tandem with others, GEIS must function smoothly as a program. If GEIS is to work as a cohesive program, it is important that its activities be well coordinated within each laboratory, between laboratories, and with the Central Hub. At some facilities that are part of GEIS, a dedicated program manager has been designated to coordinate projects. This is a valuable approach and one that should be duplicated at all facilities to the extent possible. GEIS program managers should possess expertise and experience in applied epidemiology and public health practice.

**Recommendation: The implementation of GEIS at all five overseas research laboratories and within the MHS service hubs should be coordinated by dedicated, on-site GEIS program managers who possess expertise and experience in applied epidemiology and the practice of public health.**

• Many of the facilities that are implementing GEIS projects lack an adequate number of staff possessing sufficient epidemiological expertise. As a result, some activities observed by the committee reflected incomplete incorporation of public health surveillance concepts. Infusion of epidemiological input can help ensure that GEIS concepts are clearly understood and that surveillance objectives are fully realized. The presence of a dedicated, on-site GEIS program manager who is well versed in public health and applied epidemiology is important, as mentioned above. Additional epidemiological input, on site and through the Central Hub, is also desirable.

> **Recommendation: GEIS should take steps to increase the number of personnel possessing applied epidemiological expertise available on site at laboratory facilities and within the Central Hub.**

• Current GEIS infectious disease-related training efforts (e.g., the Overseas Medical Research Laboratory Orientation Training Program) are laudable, but they are modest relative to the needs of the DoD and its public health partners and to the potential contributions of GEIS. Training professionals (including foreign national public health workers and DoD personnel) to understand, monitor, control, and prevent emerging infections is an important goal of GEIS. Providing training opportunities for U.S. civilian scientists may also prove to be a valuable use of GEIS resources. Additional investments could be made to bolster existing GEIS training activities and to develop additional, structured training programs. Training needs to be coordinated among GEIS consortium members and needs to be conducted in collaboration with public health partners (e.g., other DoD entities, the CDC, governments that host overseas laboratories, international organizations [such as the WHO], academic institutions, the Training in Epidemiology on Public Health Intervention Network [TEPHINET], and others).

> **Recommendation: GEIS's level of involvement in the training of DoD personnel, foreign national public health workers, and others should be increased.**

• Training is an extremely important but time-consuming GEIS goal. Current laboratory training activities appear to be largely project specific and do not appear to be closely coordinated within or between laboratories. Additional staffing is needed to effectively coordinate the training needs of DoD personnel, foreign national public health workers, and others.

> **Recommendation: Facilities that support GEIS and that implement training programs should be staffed to accommodate their training needs.**

• Collaboration is necessary to ensure that GEIS activities succeed, and complement and support other efforts. GEIS is actively fostering collaboration and coordination with international partners and governmental agencies in partner countries. GEIS is also taking important steps to strengthen collaborations with U.S. partner agencies, but more needs to be done to formalize these partnerships. New partnerships and means of expanding and strengthening existing partnerships can be pursued even more actively. In particular, relationships with other U.S. agencies, such as the U.S. Agency for International Development (USAID) and the CDC, need to be expanded and more closely coordinated to encourage joint planning and shared project implementation with these agencies. GEIS needs to have an identity within the global public health community such that when new initiatives related to global infectious disease surveillance and response activities are being considered by governmental and nongovernmental agencies, the potential usefulness of GEIS is considered by outside partners.

The committee notes that hiring foreign nationals to fill senior positions at overseas laboratories can benefit GEIS integration with host-country and international partners. The committee encourages the hiring of additional foreign service national personnel into senior-level positions where possible. Similarly, personnel assigned to DoD from U.S. partner agencies, such as the CDC, the National Institutes of Health, universities, and state public health agencies, can help meet staffing needs while increasing DoD ties with those agencies. The committee endorses such arrangements and encourages GEIS to actively pursue them as a means of meeting DoD staffing needs.

**Recommendation: Pursuit of collaborative, well-coordinated relationships with international organizations, U.S. government agencies (including other DoD entities), and relevant agencies of foreign governments should be continued and expanded to the extent possible. As part of these collaborations, GEIS should encourage arrangements for the sharing of staff between U.S. and international partner agencies and DoD laboratory facilities.**

• It is important that mechanisms for rapidly communicating data and other information to public health partners positioned to take action in response to an infectious disease threat be clearly identified and used. Some DoD laboratories have evolved successful communications strategies, but these mechanisms do not appear to have developed as part of a cohesive GEIS plan.

**Recommendation: In consultation with the GEIS Central Hub and collaborators, GEIS sites should prepare and act on information dissemination plans that provide for the translation of information into timely public health action.**

• Centralized data collection and analysis (as appropriate) and routine reporting of GEIS data and other information are also needed. Current methods of disseminating GEIS information are important but are insufficient. Tools such as the GEIS website (GEISWeb) and the DoD Directory of Public Health Laboratory Services can be very useful communication resources. Production of a periodic GEIS-wide publication that synthesizes GEIS information (e.g., surveillance data, progress reports, and updates on new capabilities and accomplishments) may also be appropriate.

**Recommendation: Communication of surveillance and other information within the GEIS consortium, within the DoD, to public health partners, and to the public should be improved.**

• Many of the innovative systems and techniques that GEIS is developing or encouraging, such as the DoD Directory of Public Health Laboratory Services, the Early Warning Outbreak Response System, the Electronic Surveillance System for the Early Notification of Community-Based Epidemics, and numerous others, show great promise. It is important, however, that the need for new systems and techniques be thoroughly evaluated and that plans for system development and use be clearly defined (including identification of product developers with extensive relevant expertise and experience) before projects are undertaken. Prototype systems and techniques should also be systematically evaluated before they are put to widespread use. These steps are needed to ensure that new systems and techniques contribute optimally to GEIS, to the DoD, and to global emerging infectious disease surveillance efforts.

**Recommendation: Novel surveillance systems and techniques, though potentially an important part of GEIS, should be thoroughly evaluated and plans for their development and use should be clearly defined before substantial GEIS investments in their implementation are made.**

• Periodic external review can help to determine whether the goals of GEIS are being addressed and whether those goals remain appropriate.

**Recommendation: GEIS as a whole should be subject to periodic external review (every few years) to ensure that it remains focused on its goals and that its goals remain appropriate.**

• Apart from this formal, periodic program review process, it is also essential that GEIS management (i.e., the Central Hub) has available to it clear, consistent means of routinely receiving authoritative and timely management guidance from appropriate DoD authorities as well as a means of providing feedback to appropriate DoD authorities. It is also important that there be in place within the DoD command structure clear, consistent channels through which GEIS information can be reported to achieve timely action.

**Recommendation: Clear, consistent mechanisms for providing guidance to GEIS management and channels for the reporting of GEIS information within the DoD infrastructure should be in place.**

• The committee recognizes that managing a program as diverse and diffuse as GEIS is no small task. It appears to the committee that the Central Hub is limited in its ability to effectively coordinate GEIS by a lack of administrative authority and management resources. To ensure that project guidance is acted upon, GEIS management must be positioned so that it has the authority, as well as the responsibility, to affect GEIS project implementation.

**Recommendation: GEIS management authority should be commensurate with GEIS management responsibility if program objectives are to be effectively and efficiently met.**

• GEIS would benefit from a broader, more standardized project review process (to include use of structured proposal guidelines and timelines). Reviews should incorporate input from various interested parties, such as partner agencies, overseas and MHS laboratory personnel, and other DoD representatives (e.g., Military Infectious Disease Research Program staff), as well as Central Hub staff. It may be useful to lengthen the project approval and funding cycle to allow projects to mature and to allow improved planning of new projects between reviews.

**Recommendation: Consideration should be given to revising the GEIS project review and approval process so that review and approval of GEIS projects is part of a more formally structured process—based on a set of guidelines and timelines that are clearly understood by GEIS consortium members—that includes input from individuals who represent various disciplines and interests.**

• Apart from the formal project review and approval process, Central Hub senior management staff should make additional periodic visits to the respective laboratory facilities to provide project guidance and to assess needs for assistance and opportunities for collaboration. Increased guidance from the Central Hub may help to compensate for staffing deficiencies and can foster improved coordination of GEIS projects.

**Recommendation: Staffing levels permitting, overseas and MHS-based GEIS activities should receive additional periodic assessment and guidance from the GEIS Central Hub.**

# References


AFEB (Armed Forces Epidemiology Board). 2000. AFEB Recommendations Concerning the Global Emerging Infections System (GEIS) Military Public Health Laboratory Workshop Recommendations. Memorandum for the Assistant Secretary of Defense (Health Affairs), The Surgeon General (Department of the Army), The Surgeon General (Department of the Navy), The Surgeon General (Department of the Air Force). Armed Forces Epidemiology Board, U.S. Department of Defense, Falls Church, VA, May 11, 2000. On file with the National Academies Public Access Records Office.

AFRIMS (Armed Forces Research Institute of Medical Sciences). 2000. Global Emerging Infections Surveillance and Response Systems Strategic Plan for FY00-04. Unpublished document presented to the Institute of Medicine Committee to Review the Department of Defense Global Emerging Infections Surveillance and Response System, Washington, DC, April 19, 2000.

AMSA (Army Medical Surveillance Activity). 2001. *About AMSA: DMSS.* [Online]. Available: http://amsa.army.mil/AMSA/amsa_home.htm [accessed June 19, 2001].

Ascher MS. 2000. A civilian-military virtual public health laboratory network. *Military Medicine* 165(7 Suppl. 2):1–4.

Bailey S. 1999. Policy for DoD Global, Laboratory-Based Influenza Surveillance. Memorandum for Surgeon General of the Army, Surgeon General of the Navy, Surgeon General of the Air Force, Deputy Director for Medical Readiness, J-4, the Joint Staff. U.S. Department of Defense, Health Affairs, Washington, DC, February 3, 1999. On file with the National Academies Public Access Records Office.

Bancroft WH, Schlagel C. 1997. Implementation of DoD Emerging Infectious Disease Surveillance and Response System. Memorandum for Commander, U.S. Army Medical Research and Materiel Command, Commanding Officer, U.S. Naval Medical Research and Development Command. Department of the Army, U.S. Department of Defense, Ft. Detrick, MD, June 9, 1997. On file with the National Academies Public Access Records Office.

Bolton JC, Gaydos JC. 2000. Military Public Health Laboratory Workshop Group B: A Department of Defense Directory of Public Health Laboratory Services for Infectious Agents and Public Health Laboratory System. *Military Medicine* 165(7 Suppl. 2):66–69.

Brady J, Frommelt RA. 2000. Completeness of reporting of hospitalized cases of reportable medical events, US Navy, January 1998–June 2000. *Medical Surveillance Medical Report* 6(10):17–19.

Canas LC, Lohman K, Pavlin JA, Endy T, Singh DL, Pandey P, Shrestha MP, Scott RM, Russell KL, Watts D, Hajdamowicz M, Soriano I, Douce RW, Neville J, Gaydos JC. 2000. The Department of Defense Laboratory-Based Global Influenza Surveillance System. *Military Medicine* 165(7 Suppl. 2):52–56.

CDC (U.S. Centers for Disease Control and Prevention). 1994. *Addressing Emerging Infectious Disease Threats: A Prevention Strategy for the United States*. Atlanta, GA: Centers for Disease Control and Prevention.

CDC. 1998. Preventing Emerging Infectious Diseases: A Strategy for the 21st Century. Atlanta, GA: Centers for Disease Control and Prevention.

CDC. 1999. Framework for program evaluation in public health. *Morbidity and Mortality Weekly Report* 48(RR-11):1–15.

CDC. 2000. *Draft Updated Guidelines for Evaluating Surveillance Systems—Recommendations from the Guidelines Working Group*. Atlanta, GA: Centers for Disease Control and Prevention.

Christopherson G, Baldwin TE. 1997. Department of Defense Infectious Disease Surveillance and Response System—Action Memorandum. Memorandum and attached draft for Assistant Secretary of Defense (Health Affairs). Health Affairs, U.S. Department of Defense, Washington, DC, signed March 1997. On file with the National Academies Public Access Records Office.

CISET (Committee on International Science, Engineering, and Technology). 1995. *Infectious Disease a Global Threat: Report of the National Science and Technology Council*. Working Group on Emerging and Re-emerging Infectious Disease. Washington, DC: Committee on International Science, Engineering, and Technology.

CISET. 1997. *Emerging Infectious Disease Task Force: Annual Report*. Washington, DC: Committee on International Science, Engineering, and Technology.

Cuddy J. 1997. FY 97 Budget for DoD Infectious Disease Surveillance and Response System. Memorandum for Assistant Secretary of Defense (Health Affairs), Attn: LTC Edward Baldwin, Clinical Services. Department of the Army , U.S. Department of Defense, Falls Church, VA, February 11, 1997. On file with the National Academies Public Access Records Office.

D'Amelio R, Heymann DL. 1998. Can the military contribute to global surveillance and control of infectious diseases? *Emerging Infectious Disease* 4(4):704–705.

DoS (Department of State). *Strategic Plan for International Affairs*. 1999. [Online]. Available: http://www.state.gov/www/global/general_foreign_policy/stsp828.html [accessed June 21, 2001].

Dowell S. 2001. Review of CDC's Global Infectious Disease Strategy. Memorandum to Participants in the Decatur Meeting. U.S. Centers for Disease Control and Prevention, Atlanta, GA, May 29, 2001. On file with the National Academies Public Access Records Office.

Dowell S, Levitt A, Hughes J. 2001. CDC emerging infections watch. *U.S. Medicine* 37(4):8.

Dunster L. 2001. RE: IOM Report on Kenya Lab. Personal communication to P Kelley, L Dunster, H O'Maonaigh, R Miller, E Henchal, May 22, 2001. On file with the National Academies Public Access Records Office.

Frommelt RA. 2000. Surveillance Trends: Completeness and timeliness of reporting of hospitalized notifiable cases. U.S. Army, January–June 2000. *Medical Surveillance Medical Report* 6(10):12–16.

Gambel JM, Hibbs RG Jr. 1996. U.S. military overseas medical research laboratories. *Military Medicine* 161(11):638–645.

Gardner JW, Cozzini CB, Kelley PW, Kark JA, Peterson MR, Gackstetter GD, Spencer JD. 2000. The Department of Defense Medical Mortality Registry. *Military Medicine* 165(7 Suppl. 2):57–61.

Gaydos JC. 1999. Service Hub—Military Health System Offsite Meeting Summary. Global Emerging Infections Surveillance and Response System, U.S. Department of Defense, Rockville, MD, February 23-24, 1999.

Gaydos JC. 2001a. A DoD Directory of Public Health Laboratory Services. Presentation to the Institute of Medicine Committee to Review the Department of Defense Global Emerging Infections Surveillance and Response System, March 7, 2001, Washington, DC.

Gaydos JC. 2001b. A DoD Directory of Public Health Laboratory Services and a "Virtual Public Health Laboratory (VPHL)." Unpublished paper presented to the Institute of Medicine Committee to Review the Department of Defense Global Emerging Infections Surveillance and Response System, March 7, 2001, Washington, DC.

Gaydos JC. 2001c. An Emerging Infectious Disease Alert Component for the Department of Defense (DoD) Medical Mortality Registry. Unpublished paper presented to the Institute of Medicine Committee to Review the Department of Defense Global Emerging Infections Surveillance and Response System, Washington, DC.

Gaydos JC. 2001d. Department of Defense (DoD) Laboratory-Based, Global Influenza Surveillance Program, Estimated Costs for Fiscal Year 2001. Unpublished document prepared for President, Armed Forces Epidemiology Board, July 25, 2001.

Gaydos JC. 2001e. Scope of the Program Relating to the Military Health System. Unpublished document. Department of Defense Global Emerging Infections Surveillance and Response System, Washington, DC, August 6, 2001.

GEIS (Department of Defense Global Emerging Infections Surveillance and Response System). 1998. *Addressing Emerging Infectious Disease Threats: A Strategic Plan for the Department of Defense.* Washington, DC: Walter Reed Army Institute of Research.

GEIS. 1999a. *DoD-Global Emerging Infections System—Annual Report, Fiscal Year 1999.* Unabridged. Washington, DC: Walter Reed Army Institute of Research.

GEIS. 1999b. Agenda, GEIS/OCONUS Laboratory Commanders Meeting. Global Emerging Infections Surveillance and Response System, U.S. Department of Defense, Washington, DC, May 11–14, 1999.

GEIS. 2000a. *DoD GEIS Fiscal Year 2000 Budget.* Global Emerging Infections Surveillance and Response System, U.S. Department of Defense, Washington, DC.

GEIS. 2000b. *DoD-Global Emerging Infections System—Annual Report, Fiscal Year 2000.* Unabridged. Washington, DC: Walter Reed Army Institute of Research.

GEIS. 2000c. *Fiscal Year 2001 Overall GEIS Budget Proposal.* Global Emerging Infections Surveillance and Response System, U.S. Department of Defense, Washington, DC, August 3, 2000.

GEIS. 2000d. *U.S. Army Medical Component, Armed Forces Research Institute of Medical Sciences.* [Online]. Available: http:// www.geis.ha.osd.mil [accessed December 28, 2000].

GEIS. 2000e. *U.S. Naval Medical Research Unit No. 2 (NAMRU-2).* [Online]. Available: www.geis.ha.osd.mil [accessed December 20, 2000].

GEIS. 2000f. *U.S. Naval Medical Research Unit No. 3 (NAMRU-3).* [Online]. Available: www.geis.ha.osd.mil [accessed December 28, 2000].

GEIS. 2000g. *U.S. Naval Medical Research Center, Lima (NMRCD).* [Online]. Available: www.geis.ha.osd.mil [accessed August 10, 2000].

GEIS. 2001a. *Accomplishments of the DoD-GEIS.* [Online]. Available: http://www.geis.ha.osd.mil [accessed May 31, 2001].

GEIS. 2001b. *Building a Public Health Surveillance System in the Caribbean.* [Online]. Available: http://www.geis.ha.osd.mil [accessed May 16, 2001].

GEIS. 2001c. *Department of Defense Global Emerging Infections System: Points of Contact*. Washington, DC: Walter Reed Army Institute of Research.

GEIS. 2001d. Syndromic Surveillance: A New Way To Track Emerging Infectious Diseases. [Online]. Available: http://www/getpage.asp?page=SyndromicSurveillance. htm&action=7&click=KeyProgram [accessed June 11, 2001].

GEIS. 2001e. *The DoD Worldwide Influenza Surveillance Program*. [Online].Available: http://www.geis.ha.osd.mil [accessed June 11, 2001].

GEIS. 2001f. *U.S. Naval Medical Research Unit- Kenya (USAMRU-K)*. [Online]. Available: www.geis.ha.osd.mil. [accessed June 21, 2001].

GEIS. 2001g. *U.S. Department of Defense (DoD) Initiatives*. [Online] Available: http://www.geis.ha.osd.mil [accessed March 17, 2001].

Gunzenhauser J. 2000. *MHS Army Plan FY01: Madigan AMC Surveillance Project*. Washington, DC: U.S. Department of Defense.

IOM (Institute of Medicine). 1987. *The U.S. Capacity to Address Tropical Infectious Disease Problems: Conclusions and Recommendations*. Washington, DC: National Academy Press.

IOM. 1988. *The Future of Public Health*. Washington, DC: National Academy Press.

IOM. 1992. *Emerging Infections: Microbial Threats to Health in the United States*. Washington, DC: National Academy Press.

IOM. 1999. *Strategies to Protect the Health of Deployed U.S. Forces: Medical Surveillance, Record Keeping, and Risk Reduction*. Washington, DC: National Academy Press.

IOM. 2001. *Emerging Infectious Diseases from the Global to the Local Perspective*. Workshop Summary. Washington, DC: National Academy Press.

Kalasinsky V. 2001. Directory of Public Health Laboratory Services in a Virtual Public Health Laboratory. Presentation to the Institute of Medicine Committee to Review the Department of Defense Global Emerging Infections Surveillance and Response System, March 7, 2001, Washington, DC.

Kelley P. 2000a. Building International Capacity for Emerging Infections Surveillance and Response: An Overview of the DoD global Emerging Infections System Overseas Lab Program. Presentation to the Institute of Medicine Committee to Review the Department of Defense Global Emerging Infections Surveillance and Response System, Washington, DC, April 19, 2000.

Kelley P. 2000b. Executive Summary: DoD-GEIS Influenza Surveillance—Major Impacts on 2000-2001 WHO Vaccine Recommendations. Broadcast email notice, June 30, 2000. On file with the National Academies Public Access Records Office.

Kelley P. 2001a. Building DoD's Capacity for Emerging Infections Surveillance and Response: An Orientation to the DoD-GEIS Military Health System Programs. Presentation to the Institute of Medicine Committee to Review the Department of Defense Global Emerging Infections Surveillance and Response System, San Diego, CA, January 10, 2001.

Kelley P. 2001b. Management and External Relations Overview DoD Global Emerging Infections System. Presentation to the Institute of Medicine Committee to Review the Department of Defense Global Emerging Infections and Surveillance and Response System, Washington, DC, March 7, 2001.

Kelley P. 2001c. Decision Paper: Establishing a Charter Document for the Management of DoD-GEIS. Unpublished draft paper. On file with the National Academies Public Access Records Office.

Klaucke DN, Buehler JW, Thacker SB, Parrish, RG, Trowbridge FL, Berkelman RL, The surveillance coordination group. 1988. Guidelines for evaluating surveillance systems. *Morbidity and Mortality Weekly Report* 37(Suppl 5):1–18.

Klein TA, Lee HC. 2001. Infectious Disease Surveillance for US Forces Korea (November 2000). Presentation to the Institute of Medicine Committee to Review the Department of Defense Global Emerging Infections Surveillance and Response System, San Diego, CA, January 10, 2001.

Linthicum K. 2001.*GEIS Collaborations with NASA*. Paper presented to the Institute of Medicine Committee to Review the Department of Defense Global Emerging Infections Surveillance and Response System, Washington, DC.

Lister S. 1997. Global Emerging Infections Surveillance and Response System. Memorandum for Assistant Secretary of Defense (Health Affairs). October 27, 1997. Washington, DC: Department of Defense, Department of the Army. On file with the National Academies Public Access Records Office.

Ludwig G. 2001. RE: IOM Report on Kenya Lab. Personal communication to P Kelley, L Dunster, H O'Maonaigh, R Miller, E Henchal, May 21, 2001. On file with the National Academies Public Access Records Office.

Martin E. 1997a. Surveillance and Response System for Infectious Disease. Memorandum for Assistant Secretary of the Army (Manpower and Reserve Affairs), Assistant Secretary of the Navy (Manpower and Reserve Affairs), Assistant Secretary of the Air Force (Manpower and Reserve Affairs, Installations, and Environments). Health Affairs, U.S. Department of Defense, Washington, DC, April 14, 1997. On file with the National Academies Public Access Records Office.

Martin E. 1997b. Surveillance and Response System for Infectious Disease. Memorandum for Surgeon General of the Army, Surgeon General of the Navy, Surgeon General of the Air Force. Health Affairs, U.S. Department of Defense, Washington, DC, August 21, 1997. On file with the National Academies Public Access Records Office.

Martin E. 1997c. Conditions as Executive Agent for Global Emerging Infectious Disease Surveillance and Response System (GEID&RS). Memorandum for Assistant Secretary of the Army (Manpower and Reserve Affairs). Health Affairs, U.S. Department of Defense, Washington, DC, December 9, 1997. On file with the National Academies Public Access Records Office.

Mazzuchi J. 1999. Support for P8 Funding. Memorandum for Deputy Surgeon General of the Army. Department of Defense, Health Affairs, Washington, DC, January, 19, 1999. On file with the National Academies Public Access Records Office.

McCarthy MC. 1998. FY00-05 DoD-GEIS Implementation. Commanding Officer NAMRU-3, Commanding Officer NAMRU-2, Officer in Charge NRMC-Detachment, Commander AFRIMS, Commander USAMRU-Kenya, Commander USAMRU-Brazil, Commanding Officer NMRC, Director WRAIR, November 10, 1998. On file with the National Academies Public Access Records Office.

McCarthy MC. 1999a. Goals and Objectives for FY00–05 GEIS Implementation Plan at OCONUS Medical Research Units. Memorandum to T Brewer, HV Petersen, R Rosenberg, E Antosek, P Underwood, T Sharp, M Crumrine, T Contreras, January 20, 1999. On file with the National Academies Public Access Records Office.

McCarthy MC. 1999b. FY00-05 GEIS Plan [AFRIMS]. Memorandum to T Brewer, May 19, 1999. On file with the National Academies Public Access Records Office.

McCarthy MC. 1999c. FY00-05 DoD-GEIS Plan [NAMRU-2]. Memorandum to A Corwin and HV Petersen, May 19, 1999. On file with the National Academies Public Access Records Office.

McCarthy MC. 1999d. FY00-05 DoD-GEIS Plan [NAMRU-3]. Memorandum to Eileen Villasante and Ed Antosek, May 19, 1999. On file with the National Academies Public Access Records Office.

McCarthy MC. 1999e. FY00-05 DoD-GEIS Plan [NMRCD]. Memorandum to Trueman Sharp, May 19, 1999. On file with the National Academies Public Access Records Office.

McCarthy MC. 1999f. FY00-05 DoD-GEIS Plan [USAMRU-K]. Memorandum to Ronald Rosenberg, May 19, 1999. On file with the National Academies Public Access Records Office.

McCarthy MC. 2000. FY01 DoD GEIS Funding. Memorandum to R Rosenberg, P Kelley, K Linthicum, October 16, 2000. Memorandum. On file with the National Academies Public Access Records Office.

Milhous WK, Whelen AC, Kelley PW, Kyle DE. 2000. Integrated Approaches for Elucidating Clinical and Epidemiological Relevance of Drug Resistance: Implications for Drug Development. Paper presented at the Second International Conference on Emerging Infectious Disease, Atlanta, GA.

Morrow R. 2000. *MHS Army Plan FY01: Syndromic and Sentinel Surveillance of US Navy/US Marine Corps in Support of GEIS.* Washington, DC: U.S. Department of Defense.

MIMCom (Multilateral Initiative on Malaria Communications Network). 2001. About MIM. [Online]. Available: http://www.mimcom.net [accessed June 19, 2001].

Murphy BP. 2001. *Review of Navy Environmental Health Center GEIS Activities.* Presentation to the Institute of Medicine Committee to Review the Department of Defense Global Emerging Infections Surveillance and Response System, San Diego, CA, January 9, 2001.

NAMRU-2 (U.S. Naval Medical Research Unit 2). 2000a. NAMRU2 GEIS Program. Unpublished document presented to the Institute of Medicine Committee to Review the Department of Defense Global Emerging Infections Surveillance and Response System, April 19, 2000, Washington, DC.

NAMRU-2. 2000b. U.S. Naval Medical Research Unit No. 2, Jakarta, Indonesia. Presentation to subcommittee of the Institute of Medicine Committee to Review the Department of Defense Global Emerging Infections Surveillance and Response System, Indonesia, Jakarta, October 2000.

NAMRU-2. Undated. *Early Warning Outbreak Recognition System (EWORS)—Collaboration between the Institute of Health Research and Development, Ministry of Health, Indonesia and U.S. Naval Medical Research Unit 2.*Pamphlet presented to subcommittee of the Institute of Medicine Committee to Review the Department of Defense Global Emerging Infections Surveillance and Response System, Indonesia, October 2000.

NAMRU-3 (U.S. Naval Medical Research Unit 3). 2000a. GEIS Implementation Plan at NAMRU-3, Goals and Objectives for FY00-05, Draft. Unpublished document presented to the Institute of Medicine Committee to Review the Department of Defense Global Emerging Infections Surveillance and Response System, Washington, DC, April 19, 2000.

NAMRU-3. 2000b. NAMRU-3: Cairo, Egypt. Unpublished document presented to the Institute of Medicine Committee to Review the Department of Defense Global Emerging Infections Surveillance and Response System, Washington, DC, April 19, 2000.

NIC (National Intelligence Council). 2000. *The Global Infectious Disease Threat and Its Implications for the U.S.* [Online]. Available: http://www.cia.gov/cia/publications/nic/report/nic99-17d.html [accessed: November 16, 2000].

Neville J, Canas L. 2001. *DoD-GEIS: Air Force Hub.* Presentation to the Institute of Medicine Committee to Review the Department of Defense Global Emerging Infections Surveillance and Response System, San Diego, CA, January 9, 2001.

NHRC (Naval Health Research Center). 2001a. Epidemiological Studies of Emerging Illnesses among US Military Personnel. Unpublished document presented to the Institute of Medicine Committee to Review the Department of Defense Global Emerging Infections Surveillance and Response System, San Diego, CA, January 8, 2001.

NHRC. 2001b. Review of GEIS Work by NHRC Personnel. Unpublished document presented to the Institute of Medicine Committee to Review the Department of Defense Global Emerging Infections Surveillance and Response System, San Diego, CA, January 9, 2001.

NHRC. 2001c. Naval Health Research Center Respiratory Disease Laboratory Global Emerging Infections System (GEIS). Unpublished document presented to the Institute of Medicine Committee to Review the Department of Defense Global Emerging Infections Surveillance and Response System, San Diego, CA, January 8, 2001

NIAID (National Institute of Allergy and Infectious Diseases). 1996. *Research Agenda for Emerging Infectious Diseases*. [Online]. Available: http://niaid.nih.gov/publications/execsum/contents.htm [accessed: May 13, 2001].

NIAID. 2000. *Planning for the 21st Century*. [Online] Available: http://www.niaid.nih.gov/default.htm [accessed: May 13, 2001]

NMRCD (U.S. Naval Medical Research Center Detachment). 2000a. Global Emerging Infections Surveillance Program: Five Year Strategic Plan. Unpublished document presented to the Institute of Medicine Committee to Review the Department of Defense Global Emerging Infections Surveillance and Response System, Washington, DC, April 19, 2000.

NMRCD. 2000b. Naval Medical Research Center Detachment, Lima, Peru: GEIS Program Overview. Presentation to the Institute of Medicine Committee to Review the Department of Defense Global Emerging Infections Surveillance and Response System, Lima, Peru, June 19, 2000.

NMRCD. 2000c. Overview of Naval Medical Research Center Detachment, Lima, Peru. Presentation to the Institute of Medicine Committee to Review the Department of Defense Global Emerging Infections Surveillance and Response System, Lima, Peru, June 19, 2000.

NMRCD. 2000d. U.S. Naval Medical Research Center Detachment, Lima, Peru (dated February 5, 2000). Unpublished document presented to the Institute of Medicine Committee to Review the Department of Defense Global Emerging Infections Surveillance and Response System, Lima, Peru, June 19, 2000.

NSTC (National Science and Technology Council, Executive Office of the President). 1996. *Presidential Decision Directive NSTC-7: Emerging Infections*. Washington, DC: National Science and Technology Council, Executive Office of the President.

PAHO (Pan American Health Organization). 1998. *Health in the Americas Vol. 1&2*. Washington, DC.

Pavlin JA. 2000. Bioterrorism and the importance of the public health laboratory. *Military Medicine* 165(7 Suppl. 2):25–7.

Pavlin JA. 2001a. Early Detection of Bioterrorist and Natural Disease Threats Using Syndromic Surveillance. Presentation to the Institute of Medicine Committee to Review the Department of Defense Global Emerging Infections Surveillance and Response System, San Diego, CA, January 10, 2001.

Pavlin JA. 2001b. Surveillance for Viral Respiratory Pathogens and Causes of Severe Acute Febrile Illness in Uganda. Presentation to the Institute of Medicine Committee to Review the Department of Defense Global Emerging Infections Surveillance and Response System, San Diego, CA, January 10, 2001.

Ryan D. 2000. Medical students contribute to research efforts at Navy's Peru laboratory. *Navy Medicine* (January–February):2–5.

Ryan M, Gray G, Hawksworth A, Malasig M, Hudspeth M, Poddar S. 2000. The Naval Health Research Center respiratory disease laboratory. *Military Medicine* 165(7 Suppl. 2):32–34.

Spread Spectrum Scene Online. 2001. VSAT Page. [Online]. Available: http://sss-mag.com/vsat. html [accessed: March 15, 2001].

Thornton S. 2000. MHS Army Plan FY01: Establishment of a DoD Reference Laboratory for Clinical Identification of Enteric Disease Agents. Unpublished document. Navy Environmental and Preventive Medicine Unit 5, U.S. Department of Defense, San Diego, CA.

Thornton S. 2001. Incidence, Epidemiology, and Detection of Viral Gastroenteritis Aboard U.S. Naval Vessels, A Global Emerging Infections System (GEIS) Surveillance Project. Presentation to the Institute of Medicine Committee to Review the Department of Defense Global Emerging Infections Surveillance and Response System, San Diego, CA, January 9, 2001.

USAID (U.S. Agency for International Development). 1998. *Reducing the Threat of Infectious Diseases of Major Public Health Importance.* Washington, DC: U.S. Agency for International Development.

USAID and U.S. Embassy, Lima, Peru. 2000. Strategic Objective No. 3: Improved Health, including Family Planning, of High Risk Populations. [Online]. Available: http://usembassy.state.gov/lima/wwwhasae.html[accessed August 16, 2000].

USAMRU-K. (U.S. Army Medical Research Unit, Kenya). 2000. Five-year Implementation Plan, U.S. Army Medical Research Unit–Kenya. Unpublished document presented to the Institute of Medicine Committee to Review the Department of Defense Global Emerging Infections Surveillance and Response System, April 19, 2000, Washington, DC.

Walter Reed Army Institute of Research. 1998. The New WRAIR. [Online]. Available: http://wrair-www.army.mil/welcome/newwrair.htm [accessed June 18, 2001].

Watts DM. 1996. A decade of infectious disease research. *Navy Medicine.* (July–August): 16–19.

WHO (World Health Organization). 1995. *Communicable Disease Prevention and Control: New, Emerging, and Re-Emerging Infectious Diseases.* WHA48.13. 48th World Health Assembly, agenda item 19. Geneva, Switzerland: World Health Organization.

WHO. 1996. *Emerging and Other Communicable Diseases. Strategic Plan 1996–2000.* Geneva, Switzerland: World Health Organization.

WHO. 1998. Global Infectious Disease Surveillance: Fact Sheet No. 200. June 1998. [Online]. Available: http://www.who.int/inf-fs/en/fact200.html [accessed April 20, 2001].

WHO. 1999a. *Draft: Assessment Protocol for National Communicable Disease Surveillance Systems and Epidemic Preparedness and Response Guidelines for Assessment of Teams.* Geneva, Switzerland: World Health Organization.

WHO. 1999b. *WHO Recommended Surveillance Standards,* 2nd ed. Geneva, Switzerland: World Health Organization.

WHO. 2000a. An Integrated Approach to Communicable Disease Surveillance. *Weekly Epidemiological Record* 75:1–8.

WHO. 2000b. *A Framework for Global Outbreak Alert and Response.* Geneva, Switzerland: World Health Organization.

WHO. 2000c. *WHO Report on Global Surveillance of Epidemic-Prone Infectious Diseases.* Geneva, Switzerland: World Health Organization.[Online]. Available: http://www.who.int/emc [accessed: May 14, 2001].

WHO. 2001a. Global Health Security: Epidemic Alert and Response. 107th Session, Eleventh Meeting. Geneva, Switzerland: World Health Organization.

WHO. 2001b. *Protocol for Assessment of National Communicable Disease Surveillance and Response Systems—Guidelines for Assessment Teams.* Geneva, Switzerland: World Health Organization.

Writer J. 2001a. DoD-GEIS Humanitarian Assistance Projects. Paper presented to the Institute of Medicine Committee to Review the Department of Defense Global Emerging Infections Surveillance and Response System, Washington, DC, March 7, 2001.

Writer J. 2001b. DoD-GEIS OCONUS Laboratory Training Program. Paper presented to the Institute of Medicine Committee to Review the Department of Defense Global Emerging Infections Surveillance and Response System, Washington, DC, March 7, 2001.

Writer J. 2001c. DoD-GEIS Website (GEISWeb). Paper presented to the Institute of Medicine Committee to Review the Department of Defense Global Emerging Infections Surveillance and Response System, Washington, DC, March 7, 2001.

Zajtchuk R. 1995. Implementation of a Global Surveillance Plan for Emerging Infectious Diseases Among DoD Medical Research Facilities. Memorandum for Director, Walter Reed Institute of Research, U.S. Department of Defense, August 11, 1995. On file with the National Academies Public Access Records Office.

# Appendix

# Committee Member and Staff Biographical Summaries

### Committee Members

**PHILIP S. BRACHMAN, M.D.** (Chair), is professor, Department of International Health, Rollins School of Public Health (RSPH), Emory University. He joined the Centers for Disease Control and Prevention in 1954 and worked in epidemiology and training until his retirement in 1986. He held positions in the Bureau of Epidemiology and then the Epidemiology Program Office, which he directed from 1970 to 1981. Dr. Brachman also directed the Field Epidemiology Training Program until 1986. He subsequently joined the RSPH faculty and is primarily involved in teaching regular courses in epidemiology and biostatistics in Atlanta and overseas. Dr. Brachman's current research activities include public health surveillance and nosocomial infections. He also directs the Hubert H. Humphrey Fellowship Program, a scholarship program financed by the U.S. government for foreign professionals to study and work for 1 year in the United States.

**RUTH L. BERKELMAN, M.D.,** is professor, Department of Epidemiology, Rollins School of Public Health, Emory University, with a joint appointment in the Department of International Health. Dr. Berkelman joined the Centers for Disease Control and Prevention (CDC) in 1980 as an epidemic intelligence officer, becoming director of the Division of Surveillance and Epidemiologic Studies and later directing AIDS surveillance activities for the United States. Promoted to assistant surgeon general in the U.S. Public Health Service, she was the deputy director of the

National Center for Infectious Diseases from 1992 to 1997 and then was senior adviser to the director of the CDC until 2000. She helped found the Division of Public Health of the American Society for Microbiology and currently serves on the Emerging Infections Committee of the Infectious Diseases Society of America. She is a trustee of Princeton University.

**DONALD S. BURKE, M.D.,** is professor, Department of International Health and director, Center for Immunization Research, Johns Hopkins School of Public Health. Previously he worked at the Walter Reed Army Institute of Research, where he served as chief of the Department of Virus Diseases and Director of the Division of Retrovirology. He has also served as director for the U.S. Military HIV/AIDS Research Program and chief of the Department of Virology for the Armed Forces Research Institute of Medical Sciences in Bangkok, Thailand. His interests include the control of human epidemic viral diseases, the study of tropical viral diseases such as dengue and encephalitis, molecular epidemiology, and the evolution of human viruses. He served on the National Research Council's (NRC's) Roundtable for the Development of Drugs and Vaccines Against AIDS and is past president of the American Society of Tropical Medicine. Dr. Burke recently chaired the NRC Committee on Climate, Ecosystems, Infectious Diseases, and Human Health.

**KATHLEEN F. GENSHEIMER, M.D., M.P.H.,** is state epidemiologist, Bureau of Health, Maine Department of Human Services. Previously she served as an epidemic intelligence officer with the Centers for Disease Control and Prevention and as a commissioned corps officer in the U.S. Public Health Service. She was a member of the executive committee of the Council of State and Territorial Epidemiologists from 1989 to 1999 and served as secretary of that organization from 1993 to 1999. She was the chair of the American Society for Microbiology's Public Health Division Y in 2000. Dr. Gensheimer currently serves as a consultant to the Interagency Group on Influenza Pandemic Preparedness, U.S. Department of Health and Human Services (DHHS); as a member of the National Advisory Council for the Elimination of Tuberculosis, DHHS; and as a member of the Emerging Infections Committee, Infectious Diseases Society of America.

**C. JAMES HOSPEDALES, M.B. B.S., F.F.P.H.M., E.I.S.,** is director, Caribbean Epidemiology Center, Pan American Health Organization, World Health Organization (West Indies). Dr. Hospedales has extensive experience in the surveillance and control of disease, in the United Kingdom, the United States, and the Caribbean. He has extensive experience in the planning, implementation, and evaluation of national and international surveillance systems (e.g., physician sentinels, laboratory networks, and human immunodeficiency virus infection/AIDS). He has served as the leader of team investigations of outbreaks of cholera in Guyana (1992) and Legionnaires' disease in Antigua (1996) and as chairman of the Caribbean Workshop on Control and Elimination of Leprosy in Trinidad (1991) and has provided disease surveillance following hurricanes Hugo (1989) and Luis and Marilyn (1996), the volcanic eruption at Montserrat (1995), and the flood disaster in Guyana (1996). He also participated in the World Health Organization Consultation on Epidemiologic and Statistical Methods of Rapid Health Assessment, held in Geneva, Switzerland, in 1990.

**ANN MARIE KIMBALL, M.D., M.P.H., F.A.C.P.,** is associate professor, Health Services and Epidemiology, Adjunct in Medicine, University of Washington. She also serves as the director and graduate program coordinator, M.P.H. Program, School of Public Health and Community Medicine, University of Washington. Dr. Kimball has devoted her career to studying health issues and has worked in numerous positions in the United States and abroad. Her research interests are primarily in international health, trade, human immunodeficiency virus (HIV) infection/AIDS, emerging infections, maternal and child health, and health informatics. She has previously served as a member of the Institute of Medicine Forum on Emerging Infections, as a member of the Department of Health Emerging and Reemerging Diseases Strategic Planning Task Force, as regional adviser for the Pan American Health Organization in HIV infection/AIDS, and as the chair of the National Alliance of State and Territorial AIDS Directors in the United States. She has served as a U.S. delegate to the American Pacific Economic Council Industry, Science & Technology Working Group.

**GUÉNAËL R. RODIER, M.D.,** is director, Department of Communicable Disease Surveillance and Response, World Health Organization (WHO; Geneva, Switzerland). His work experience also includes service at the International Health Program, University of Maryland at Baltimore, and as an infectious disease epidemiologist, U.S. Naval Medical Research Unit 3 (Cairo, Egypt). Dr. Rodier possesses disease-specific experience in filovirus hemorrhagic fevers (caused by Ebola, Marburg, and Rift Valley fever viruses), human immunodeficiency virus infection/AIDS, cholera, dengue, hantavirus infection, and many others. He has been actively involved in the development of new WHO strategies and tools for communicable disease surveillance; has led and managed medical teams in private practice, the U.S. Navy, and the WHO; and has coordinated international field teams conducting research projects, outbreak investigations, and assessments of national surveillance systems.

**RONALD K. ST. JOHN, M.D., M.P.H.,** is executive director, Center for Emergency Preparedness and Response, Health Canada, and associate professor of medicine, University of Ottawa Medical School. Dr. St. John has also served as a commissioned officer in the U.S. Public Health Service, as the deputy director of the National AIDS Program Office, and as a program coordinator for the Health Situation and Trend Assessment Program, Pan American Health Organization. He is a member of the American Association for the Advancement of Science, the American Public Health Association, the International Epidemiology Association, and the Commissioned Officers Association, among others. Dr. St. John has received many honors and awards, including the Pan American Health Organization Medal for Outstanding Management and the U.S. Public Health Service Distinguished Service Medal. He is also a member of the Canadian Committee to Advise on Tropical Medicine and Travel and the Committee to Plan the HIV/AIDS Satellite Prevention Conference for the XIth International Conference on AIDS.

## Study Staff

**RICHARD N. MILLER, M.D., M.P.H.,** is director, Medical Follow-Up Agency, Institute of Medicine. He possesses an extensive background in preventive medicine and military medicine and has served as public health officer in the Canal Zone, Republic of Panama; in Thailand; and in Germany; as well as serving as director, Division of Preventive Medicine, Walter Reed Army Institute of Research (WRAIR). Dr. Miller is a member of numerous professional societies and is also a member of the General Preventive Medicine Residency Advisory Committee, WRAIR.

**HEATHER C. O'MAONAIGH** has served as a staff member with the Institute of Medicine since 1998. She holds a master's degree in demography from Georgetown University and a bachelor of science in sociology from Western Washington University.